11/14

What's Wrong with the Poor?

STUDIES IN SOCIAL MEDICINE

Allan M. Brandt, Larry R. Churchill, and
Jonathan Oberlander, *editors*

What's Wrong with the Poor?

PSYCHIATRY, RACE, AND THE WAR ON POVERTY

Mical Raz

THE UNIVERSITY OF NORTH CAROLINA PRESS
Chapel Hill

*Research for this book
was supported by the
Polonsky Academy for
Advanced Study in the
Humanities and Social
Sciences at the Van Leer
Jerusalem Institute.*

39.95

Designed and set in Arno Pro by Rebecca Evans

The paper in this book meets the guidelines for permanence
and durability of the Committee on Production Guidelines
for Book Longevity of the Council on Library Resources.

The University of North Carolina Press has been a member
of the Green Press Initiative since 2003.

Library of Congress Cataloging-in-Publication Data
Raz, Mical.
What's wrong with the poor? : psychiatry, race, and the
war on poverty / Mical Raz.
p. ; cm.—(Studies in social medicine)
Includes bibliographical references and index.
ISBN 978-1-4696-0887-7 (hardback)
1. United States—Social policy. 2. Poor—Government
policy—United States. 3. Poor—United States. 4. Poverty—
Psychological aspects—United States. 5. Deprivation
(Psychology) I. Title. II. Series: Studies in social medicine.
[DNLM: 1. Poverty—history—United States. 2. Poverty—
psychology—United States. 3. African Americans—
history—United States. 4. Cultural Deprivation—United
States. 5. History, 20th Century—United States. 6. Public
Policy—history—United States. HC 79.P6]
HV95.R39 2013
362.50973—dc23   2013015589

17 16 15 14 13   5 4 3 2 1

To the brave MEN *and* WOMEN—
PATIENTS, STAFF, *and* VOLUNTEERS—
at Physicians for Human Rights, Israel

CONTENTS

ILLUSTRATIONS

ACKNOWLEDGMENTS

IT IS A GREAT PLEASURE to acknowledge the many people who have supported me throughout this project. I began this research while a Polonsky Postdoctoral Fellow at the Van Leer Jerusalem Institute in 2009. I am grateful to Gabriel Motzkin and the administrative staff who supported my work and my archival research. As a historian of American psychiatry working in Israel, I had the good fortune to benefit from a small but strong community. Otniel Dror suggested the topic of sensory deprivation; conversations with Eduardo Duniec, Noah Efron, and Michael Zakim helped shape my early ideas. My longtime mentor, José Brunner, has always encouraged me to pay attention to the politics of mental health. Rona Cohen offered wise insights and unwavering support.

At Yale University, I was incredibly lucky to join the vibrant history of medicine community. My primary debt is to my postdoctoral mentor, Naomi Rogers, who gave generously of her time and wisdom and guided me through the different stages of writing and editing this book. While encouraging me to find a more narrative tone, Naomi helped me ground my ideas in American history. Equally important, Naomi provided a role model for being a politically engaged historian, a feminist, and a dedicated educator. I am also grateful to John Warner, who welcomed me to the department and supported my work and professional development. Participants at the Holmes Workshop offered valuable feedback on my work. I am particularly grateful to Ziv Eisenberg, Kate Irving, Rodion Kosovsky, Marco Ramos, Sally Romano, and Courtney Thompson from the Yale History of Psychiatry Working Group and the Program in the History of Science and Medicine. Debbie Doroshow, who read and commented on early versions of this book, has been a long-time supporter and wise colleague. Matthew Gambino served as an invaluable sounding board in discussing the intersections of race, psychiatry, and poverty. Ewa Lech and Ramona Moore provided me with endless technical and administrative support, useful advice, and kindness.

Historians of American medicine provided a valuable community within which to develop my ideas and arguments. I am particularly grateful to Andrea Tone for her continued support and friendship. Conversations with Jonathan Metzl provided inspiration in analyzing the race riots. Gerald Oppenheimer, David Rosner, and the other participants in the Rosner Lecture Series at the Columbia University Department of Sociomedical Sciences, where I presented an early version of chapter 3, provided thoughtful comments, drawing my attention not only to what I was saying but to what was being heard.

In the course of my research, I was fortunate to have the assistance of knowledgeable and accommodating archivists. I am particularly grateful to Lizette Royer Barton and Dorothy Gruich at the University of Akron Center for the History of Psychology; Diane Richardson at the Oskar Diethelm Library, Cornell University; Shelley Sweeney at the University of Manitoba; Gary McMillan at the American Psychiatry Association; Bryan Whitledge at the University of Illinois at Urbana-Champaign; and Stephen Greenberg at the National Institutes of Health. The Hamilton Grant from the University of Manitoba and the J. R. Kantor Award from the Center for the History of Psychology at the University of Akron helped fund research travel from Israel.

At the University of North Carolina Press, I had the good fortune to work with Joe Parsons, who enthusiastically pushed this project forward. Having such a skilled, accessible, and kind editor made the publishing process seem simple. Barbara Beatty and Gerald Grob, who reviewed the book manuscript, offered astute insights.

Friends and family have provided love, support, and dog-sitting assistance over the years and across continents. Noga and Neri Minsky welcomed me to their home during my numerous research trips to the East Coast. Mentors and colleagues at the Internal Medicine J Department at the Tel Aviv Medical Center have been patient, kind, and often awe-inspiring.

My biggest debt is to my parents. While my father, Tzvi, died two years before I began this project, there is much of him evident throughout the book. He loved history, was strongly committed to justice, and cherished the rather romantic notion that education could combat poverty. I am grateful for his insistence that I study medicine, which he thought would at the very least keep me out of trouble. All of my childhood memories of my mother,

Orna, involve books and letters, yet she always prioritized community action and social solidarity over formal education. She and her partner, Johnny, have provided love and encouragement throughout this project. Finally, I am grateful to Sophie, whose infinite furry wisdom helped me never lose sight of the truly important things in life.

What's Wrong with the Poor?

INTRODUCTION

AT A WHITE HOUSE AFTERNOON TEA in February 1965, Lady Bird Johnson announced the establishment of Project Head Start, an early childhood
educational program that would serve children—many of them African
American—from low-income homes. Designed and administered by the
Office of Economic Opportunity, this new program drew much media attention. Moved by the educational opportunities these children would be
afforded but distressed at their meager backgrounds, the First Lady described
how some of these children had never seen a flower, had never sat in a chair;
some did not even know their own names.[1]

Today, these clearly erroneous perceptions of children from low-income
and minority backgrounds seem misguided, even comical. Why would a
well-intentioned public figure such as the First Lady display such a negative
perception of children from low-income homes? What did she think their
homes were like—isolated dungeons? As a matter of fact, she did, and she
expected many of her listeners to think the same way. Images of extreme isolation shaped the prevailing perception of the family life in low-income homes,
and throughout the 1960s, politicians and child mental health experts alike
viewed the lives of low-income children and their parents through a focus on
what was missing. Relying on experimental research and infant-observation
studies, liberal policymakers and mental health experts alike were confident
in their knowledge that the poor had very little indeed.

Much of the expert knowledge that provided the scientific basis of this
view of low-income homes was derived from experiments in sensory deprivation. These experiments, first carried out in the laboratory of eminent psychologist Donald O. Hebb at McGill University in Montreal, were designed
to examine the effects of reduced external stimulation on behavior, cognitive
ability, and psychological makeup. Differing in protocol and methods, these
experiments shared the goal of reducing external stimuli, an objective that

defined them as belonging to an emerging field of scientific inquiry. Donning goggles, earmuffs, and mittens, subjects spent hours and even days in dark, empty rooms. Before and after the experiment, they completed memory and learning tests and psychological evaluations.

Hebb had long been interested in the effects of the environment on the brain. His 1936 doctoral dissertation, advised by psychologist Karl Lashley, examined the learning abilities of rats raised in complete darkness. Upon graduation, Hebb took on different junior research posts that led him away from his original research interests. He cobbled together a position as a research assistant at Harvard and later worked with pioneering neurosurgeon Wilder Penfield at the Montreal Neurological Institute. Hebb evaluated Penfield's postoperative patients to define the cognitive and psychological effects of brain surgery. In 1942, Hebb accepted a research position at the Yerkes Primate Lab in Florida, where he carried out psychological and cognitive assessments of primates.[2] There he worked alongside experimental psychologist Austin Riesen, who examined the development of chimpanzees raised in darkness, and became a leading expert on deprivation experiments in animals.[3] In 1947, Hebb was appointed professor of psychology at McGill University, and he remained there for most of his career. His interest in the interaction between environment and neurological development and his experience in assessing cognitive and psychological abilities culminated in his widely influential 1949 monograph, *The Organization of Behavior*.[4] Proposing an innovative theory of behavior, Hebb's work was unique in its focus on how the environment and past experiences shaped neural connections. In a continuation of this study, as professor of psychology at McGill, Hebb embarked on a series of experiments examining animals raised in enriched or restricted environments. In the early 1950s, Hebb started examining the effects of restricted environments on adult human volunteers, and this research became caught up in government intelligence concerns.[5]

In June 1951, Hebb, as chair of the Human Relations and Research Committee of the Canadian Defence Research Boards, met with senior researcher Cyril Haskins of the U.S. Central Intelligence Agency; Ormond Solandt, chair of the Canadian Defence Research Board; and other leading Canadian scientists. At this meeting, Hebb suggested that by sensory deprivation, the "individual could be led into a situation whereby ideas, etc. might be implanted."[6] Hebb later publicly recalled that the work at McGill University began "with the problem of brainwashing." Although "we were not permitted to say so in the first publishing," he explained, the "chief impetus" for this research "was the dismay at the kind of 'confessions' being produced at the Russian Communist trials."[7] Scientists and intelligence officials saw sensory deprivation research as having the potential to explain extreme cases of changes in attitude, in particular, false confessions and "brainwashing." From 1951 to 1954, Hebb received funding from the Canadian Defence Research Board for his research on sensory deprivation.[8]

At first, Hebb's results were kept secret despite his concerns about academic competition, as other researchers began examining similar questions of the effect of environmental restriction. Hebb and his team presented their preliminary, classified results at the Defence Research Board's 1952 symposium. Their subjects suffered from hallucinations, delusions, disorientation, and out-of-body experiences and scored lower in solving mathematic problems. As part of the research protocol, subjects were asked before the experiment about their attitudes toward controversial topics such as the evolutionary theory or the existence of psychic phenomena. They then underwent sensory deprivation and were subsequently played recordings of arguments against the views they had previously voiced. Testing indicated that they responded more positively than before. Thus, sensory deprivation rendered the subjects more susceptible to attempts to induce attitude change.[9] Hebb and his team had found an extremely powerful tool.

Only in 1954, after descriptions of these studies were leaked to the popular press, was Hebb granted permission to report his results to the scientific community.[10] Early results published in the *Canadian Journal of Psychology* were prefaced by a cover story that explained that these experiments were designed to shed light on "the lapses of attention that may occur when a man must give close and prolonged attention to some aspect of an environment in which nothing is happening." Examples included "watching a radar screen hour after hour" or "inexplicable" highway accidents; no mention was made of attempts to induce a change of attitude.[11]

This article was the first of a series of publications on experiments involving what would become known as sensory deprivation, which were carried out with human subjects. These pioneering experiments were further developed by researchers in laboratories across North America, including notable researchers such as psychoanalyst and expert in dolphin studies John Lilly at the National Institutes of Health, psychiatrist Philip Solomon at Harvard, and John Zubek at the University of Manitoba. Hebb's students—for example, Maitlin Baldwin at the National Institute of Mental Health and Canadian psychologist Ronald Melzack, who later credited his interest in the study of

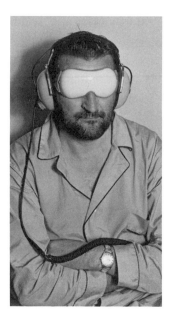

University of Manitoba researcher
John Zubek outside his sensory
deprivation chamber, ca. 1966.
Photo by David Portigal. Conserved
in the John Zubek Collection,
University of Manitoba Archives
and Special Collections, Winnipeg.

pain to observations he had made during Hebb's early sensory deprivation experiments with dogs—went on to assume leading positions in sensory deprivation research.[12] Within seven years of Hebb's team's first publication, more than 230 articles on sensory deprivation appeared in leading scientific journals, and most of the authors cited Hebb's work. In 1958, Harvard University held a symposium on sensory deprivation funded indirectly by the intelligence community.[13] It attracted leading researchers who approached the topic from diverse backgrounds: psychiatrists, research psychologists, physiologists, and the director of research at the U.S. Air Force's Aerospace Medical Laboratory. Their papers encompassed a wide range of interests, from the use of sensory deprivation to facilitate psychotherapeutic intervention to changes in EEG patterns that could be documented during isolation.[14] Whereas the late 1940s had seen only a handful of researchers working on the effects of a restricted environment on animals, the interest in sensory deprivation sparked by the McGill studies also led to a surge in animal research in the late 1950s and early 1960s. Researchers across North America experimented with rats, cats, dogs, and primates in restricted and enriched environments, assessing the effects of sensory deprivation.[15] Thus, while both animal studies and the military interests of the United States and Canada influenced the trajectory of sensory deprivation research into the study of human volunteers, this trajectory in turn led to further research on experimental animals.

At the height of its popularity, sensory deprivation was invoked as explanation for a wide range of phenomena from various fields. Psychologists and psychiatrists published articles in professional journals speculating on the role of sensory deprivation in accounts of shipwrecked sailors and Arctic explorers as well as in more mundane situations, such as accidents involving long-distance truck drivers.[16] Well-documented clinical phenomena were also subject to this reinterpretation. Patients often suffered from hallucinations following ophthalmologic surgery; the eye patch was faulted for causing visual deprivation, a form of sensory deprivation. This belief led to a questioning of the necessity of prolonged patching and a change in postoperative care on ophthalmologic services.[17] Psychotic episodes following surgery and immobilization were reinterpreted as caused by sensory deprivation.[18]

Even the success of the psychoanalytic setting was credited to sensory deprivation. Psychoanalyst Karl Menninger used the framework of sensory deprivation experiments to describe how psychoanalysis induced regression. One psychoanalyst ventured that the "technical conditions of psychoanalysis—the couch, the injunction against 'acting out,' the psychoanalyst as a blank screen, etc—involve stimulus deprivation." Similarly, another analyst suggested that the "quiet of the analyst's office, the patient's supine position, his inability to see the analyst and the absence of everyday verbal response" created a form of sensory deprivation.[19]

Sensory deprivation experiments provided the impetus for a reevaluation of popular mental health theories, leading researchers to rethink their work through an emphasis on what was missing. The field enjoyed both significant scientific prestige and wide cultural currency, as a number of popular articles in the mid-1950s described the psychological perils of monotony, boredom, and isolation.[20] By the early 1960s, this emphasis on deprivation became the leading theoretical approach in the American mental health profession.

As this book demonstrates, mental health experts privileged interpretations that focused on what was missing in contexts as diverse as children in orphanages to the race riots of the 1960s. *What's Wrong with the Poor?* examines how this deprivation discourse of mental health and child development experts shaped social policy in the 1960s. Sensory deprivation serves as the starting point for this analysis, which follows how theories of deprivation developed by psychiatrists and psychologists became the leading framework by which to evaluate the lives, needs, and abilities of low-income children and adults of color. Various external stimuli were seen to be crucial for the development of normal intelligence and a healthy psyche. While sensory deprivation experiments were based on extreme laboratory conditions in which subjects were isolated and deprived of nearly all external stimulation, the findings from these experiments were seen to be applicable to situations far more mundane. From descriptions of gray, drab buildings in the urban ghetto to what kind of toys offered the most stimulation to toddlers, far-reaching interpretations of early sensory deprivation experiments were invoked by mental health professionals and child development experts to explain a wide range of phenomena.

Most of the questions addressed through the framework of deprivation, however, were about two overlapping sections of American society—poor and black. The poor had less; African Americans, disproportionately represented among America's poor, were seen to have practically nothing. New theories and terms were developed to describe what low-income and mainly African American families were seen as lacking, and the theory of "cultural deprivation" gained wide currency. A particular emphasis was placed on children, who could be targeted with early preventative intervention, and services were set up to provide them with what they were seen to be lacking: nutritious food, stimulating toys and books, trips to museums, and ultimately nursery teachers who could fulfill the role of middle-class mothers. The children's parents were targeted by in-home intervention programs that offered instruction in what were seen to be more effective parenting techniques. *What's Wrong with the Poor?* examines the historical origins of the deprivation hypothesis and argues that "cultural deprivation" was based on race- and class-specific interpretations of sensory and maternal deprivation. It examines how the highly political term "cultural deprivation" became the leading framework by which to conceptualize the needs and challenges of children from low-income and minority homes. Yet this process was not inevitable: A particular political and cultural context led child mental health experts, educators, and policymakers to embrace the deprivation theory and its translation into social policy.

By the late 1960s, a number of influential critiques of the cultural deprivation approach had been published or presented at leading conferences. By emphasizing the pathological home and family life of individuals from low-income backgrounds, critiques of the cultural deprivation approach argued that this theory was a method of shifting responsibility onto the poor, or blaming the victim, as psychologist William Ryan argued. In the 1950s and 1960s, liberal social scientists and policymakers embraced theories of racial difference that focused on perceived damage or deficits. By the 1970s, however, these same cultural deprivation approaches were often deemed racist.[21] What had been the bon ton of racial liberals and antiracist scholars soon became seen as the purview of racial conservatives and even racists. From the mid-1970s onward, the term "cultural deprivation" fell into disuse, and it has been replaced by descriptions referring solely to socioeconomic status.

From widespread acceptance to complete disavowal in less than a decade and a half, deprivation theory did not go from right to wrong; no new data were found to disprove its basic assumptions. It was inextricably linked to the political atmosphere of the 1960s and provided the scientific rationale for federal interventions. *What's Wrong with the Poor?* examines the interplay between psychiatric theory and social policy, analyzing how the discourse of experts influenced public policy and was reflected in the discourse of politicians. Theories of deprivation became the main currency for an exchange of ideas, fostering professional cooperation between mental health experts and liberal-minded policymakers.

Deprivation theory provided the basis for numerous federally funded interventions, including Project Head Start, which has served more than twenty-five million American children since it was established as a summer intervention program in 1965.[22] A palatable theoretical framework by which to conceptualize funding priorities that might otherwise have raised objections among racial and social conservatives, deprivation theory facilitated the acceptance of antipoverty interventions. It also, however, has had a long-lasting effect on American culture and has profoundly shaped how both health professionals and educators view children from low-income and culturally and linguistically diverse homes. Focusing on what is missing rather than what is there, on deprivation rather than on differences or strengths and coping mechanisms, deprivation theory has left a legacy from which current educators are working hard to distance themselves. *What's Wrong with the Poor?* examines an important chapter in American social policy and provides a provocative analysis of liberal politics.

Chapter 1 examines how theories of sensory deprivation led to a reevaluation of the accepted psychological theory of maternal deprivation, as experts, including psychologist Mary Ainsworth and psychoanalyst René Spitz, debated whether maternal care was unique or simply a form of environmental stimulation. This tension between sensory and maternal deprivation was ultimately resolved through a class-specific interpretation of deprivation. Children from middle-class homes were seen to be at risk for maternal deprivation when placed in day care facilities and separated from their presumably competent mothers, while day care for children from low-income and mostly minority families was seen to be therapeutic, ostensibly countering the sensory deprivation the children suffered in their inadequate homes. Depriving for the middle class, therapeutic for the deprived, this deprivation discourse was reflected in President Richard M. Nixon's 1971 veto of a bill that would have provided universal day care, and it remains evident in current American day care policy.

Chapter 2 critically examines the concept of cultural deprivation, arguing that it was based on race- and class-specific interpretations of better-established forms of deprivation—nutritional, maternal, and sensory deprivation. There were no empiric data on cultural deprivation; rather, researchers uncritically cited sensory deprivation experiments and psychologists' infant observations, using maternal and sensory deprivation as proof of cultural deprivation. "Slum" homes of poor black urban families were seen to cause sensory deprivation, whereas the "matriarchal" structure of African American families, famously referred to by Daniel P. Moynihan in "The Negro Family: The Case for National Action" (1965) as pathological, was somewhat counter-intuitively seen to cause "maternal deprivation." The second half of the chapter examines the debate that followed the 1969 publication of hereditarian psychologist Arthur Jensen's critique of compensatory education, in which he first articulated his theory of the hereditary component of intelligence. Both Jensen and his detractors relied on different interpretations of deprivation theories; the chapter examines how these theories were enlisted to further both sides of the nature-nurture debate.

The translation of deprivation into practical intervention programs targeting children from low-income African American homes is the focus of chapter 3. Although ostensibly targeting cultural deprivation, these programs explicitly attempted to counter the perceived sensory deprivation caused by the "impoverished environment" of poor black homes as well as maternal deprivation attributed to inadequate mothers. The chapter evaluates compensatory education programs developed in the early 1960s and then turns to Mobilization for Youth, a community action program active in the early and mid-1960s on Manhattan's Lower East Side. The program targeted mainly minorities and at the time was considered radical, as it supported community leaders in controversial struggles such as a rent strike protesting tenement conditions and demands for an investigation into accusations of police misconduct. Yet even this seemingly radical program was based on theories of deprivation that shaped the forms of intervention offered. The chapter ends by examining two key moments in Project Head Start: its establishment and its proponents' response to early unfavorable evaluations. The chapter demonstrates how programs designed to combat cultural deprivation focused on providing sensory stimulation and surrogate "maternal care" to compensate for perceived deprivations in those areas.

Theories of deprivation profoundly changed how mental health experts and childhood educators viewed intellectual disability. Chapter 4 examines how deprivation became an accepted etiological factor for intellectual disability, appearing in all the major classifications of the time and readily adopted by psychiatrists. Theories of deprivation helped shift the focus from the profoundly disabled to the large group of children who were diagnosed at the time with "mild mental retardation." Yet by the mid-1960s, "mild mental retardation" became a category used to diagnose primarily African American children from low-income homes, as "cultural deprivation"—a virtual synonym for being black and poor—became accepted as a cause of intellectual disability. The chapter examines how theories of deprivation provided the scientific framework that enabled the diagnoses of a disproportionately large number of African American children as "mildly mentally retarded."

Chapter 5 examines how growing concerns regarding the violence and psychological detachment that were seen to characterize predominantly black inner cities provided the impetus for the development of environmental psychology in the era of white flight. Theories of the dangers of urban living drew heavily on early sensory deprivation experiments; accordingly, "slums"—depicted as gray, windowless, unstimulating—were seen to be depriving. In the midst of the militant Black Power stage of civil rights movement, and particularly following the outbreak of urban riots throughout the United States, a special emphasis was placed on the role of slum conditions in the genesis of urban violence. The chapter examines the urban race riots of the 1960s, focusing on the deliberations and final report of National Advisory Commission on Civil Disorders.

The conclusion asks how the mental health profession can help the poor without pathologizing them. Instead of examining the structural causes of poverty and inequality, experts too often focus on perceived individual character flaws or psychiatric deficits. Deprivation theory remains very much alive in American culture, peering from behind seemingly race- and class-neutral adjectives. The book concludes with a call for a closer evaluation of how psychiatric theories are used to shape public policy.

CHAPTER ONE

A Mother's Touch?

From Deprivation to Day Care

IN 1950, EMINENT BRITISH PSYCHOANALYST John Bowlby was appointed as a short-term consultant to the World Health Organization on the subject of homeless children in post–World War II Europe. This position proved to be a turning point in his career. Bowlby, who had previously conducted research on the impact of children's separation from their mothers or mother-substitutes early in life, had a long-standing interest in what he later came to call deprivation.[1] Drawing from the available research on children in institutions as well as his own findings, he prepared his report, *Maternal Care and Mental Health*, published in 1951. It was "essential for mental health," Bowlby argued, that "the infant and young child should experience a warm, intimate, and continuous relationship with his mother (or mother-substitute) in which both find satisfaction and enjoyment." If this relationship was absent or insufficient—what Bowlby termed "maternal deprivation"—serious consequences for the child's future mental health and character development would ensue.[2] An adapted version of the report appeared in 1953 as *Child Care and the Growth of Love*, quickly becoming a best seller, and the volume was reprinted six times within ten years and translated into fourteen languages.[3] Bowlby, at the time the deputy director of the Tavistock Clinic in London, became a household name on both sides of the Atlantic, and American newspapers closely followed his research findings.[4] Although Bowlby himself had referred to mothers or "mother-substitutes," his work further perpetuated traditional gender roles. Later critics have characterized Bowlby's work as a reactionary theory designed to pressure women into staying at home with their children for fear of risking serious health consequences.[5] Bowlby's insistence on the crucial role of mothers while ignoring a whole spectrum of other possible factors led British psychoanalyst and feminist Juliet Mitchell to quip that "evacuee children were 'maternally deprived'—bombs and poverty and absent fathers didn't come into it."[6]

"Maternal deprivation" rapidly gained currency among American mental health and child development experts. Bowlby's report had surveyed the work of prominent American researchers, most notably psychoanalytically trained psychiatrists René Spitz and David Levy. The popularization of maternal deprivation in the early 1950s drew further attention to these studies and provided the scientific impetus for subsequent observation studies of infants designed to elucidate the wide-reaching detrimental effects of this form of deprivation.[7]

Concurrently, concepts of sensory deprivation had increasingly become popular and were used to describe a wide spectrum of phenomena. This focus on the necessity of sensory stimulation for normal early development soon led mental health experts to reexamine theories that highlighted the dangers of maternal deprivation. Experimental psychologists, basing their hypotheses on animal experimentation, questioned the accepted view of mother love as the crucial component in normal infant development. Instead, they proposed that a lack of sensory stimulation was the immediate cause of psychological damage. Conversely, psychoanalytically oriented researchers in the field of maternal deprivation cited findings of sensory deprivation experiments as proof of the necessity of maternal care. Thus blossomed a new cooperation between psychologists and child development experts from entirely different theoretic backgrounds. While many welcomed this interdisciplinary cooperation, other psychoanalytically inclined experts expressed concern at attempts to replace the abstract concept of mothering with specific variables of sensory stimulation. Some researchers viewed the two theories as complementary, commenting on the potential for mutual benefit from reliance on insight gleaned from different theoretical and experimental approaches. In their 1963 book, *Growth Failure in Maternal Deprivation*, pediatricians Robert L. Patton and Lytt I. Gardner devoted the entire first chapter to the topic of sensory deprivation and its relationship to maternal deprivation, voicing their hope that "scientists in biology and in the behavioral sciences might find useful this study of the organic manifestations of" maternal deprivation, which they called "a special form of sensory deprivation."[8]

Here, I analyze the adoption of the basic premises, experimental methods, and terminology of sensory deprivation research into maternal deprivation theory. I examine how leading figures in the field of maternal deprivation—most notably, Mary Ainsworth and René Spitz—gradually accepted the sensory deprivation theory. I then evaluate the practical implications of the interrelations between theories of sensory and maternal deprivation as they are demonstrated in debates over day care in the United States. An economically stratified approach to deprivation emerged—middle-class children in day care programs were seen to be at risk for maternal deprivation, while day care programs targeting low-income and minority children were seen as therapeutic, combating sensory deprivation, and not carrying the risk of maternal deprivation. I conclude by analyzing President Nixon's 1971 veto of a bill designed to provide universal day care, which exemplifies the tension between maternal and sensory deprivation and demonstrates how these concepts were applied selectively according to race and class. While the following chapters deal with racialized views of deprivation that emerged in the early and mid-1960s, this chapter focuses mainly on socioeconomic biases in the controversy over whether maternal deprivation was simply one form of sensory deprivation or was a unique psychological phenomenon.

Maternal Deprivation Theorists
Respond to Sensory Deprivation

Psychologist Mary Salter Ainsworth was one of the most influential figures in maternal deprivation research. After receiving her doctorate from the University of Toronto in 1939, Mary Salter served in the Canadian Women's Corps, obtaining the rank of major. She then joined the psychology department faculty at her alma mater and pursued research on psychological testing and Rorschach evaluations. Newly married in 1950, she followed her husband, an army veteran and graduate student in her department, to London, where he completed his doctorate. Although Ainsworth's dissertation had examined children's sense of security, she had never been particularly interested in psychoanalysis. Yet an advertisement in the London *Times* led her to a research position at the Tavistock Clinic, where she worked with John Bowlby on a project examining the effects of maternal deprivation. Upon Leonard Ainsworth's graduation, Mary Ainsworth followed her husband to Uganda, where she spent two years performing observations on mother-infant interactions. In 1955, Leonard Ainsworth's work took the couple to Baltimore, where Mary Ainsworth worked her way from an adjunct position involving psychological testing and clinical supervision to professor of development psychology at Johns Hopkins University. Following a painful divorce in 1960, Mary Ainsworth never remarried and had no children of her own.[9] Much of her remarkable career was devoted to the evaluation of mother-infant relations, and she became a pioneer in the nascent field of attachment theory, examining how the interactions between infants and parents shaped lifelong psychological relations. Ainsworth worked closely with Bowlby throughout her career, considering him a mentor, and shared his perceptions of the necessity of maternal care. The two corresponded and collaborated until Bowlby's death in 1990, and their letters provide valuable insight into how the main proponents of maternal deprivation viewed the emerging field of sensory deprivation and how this view changed over time.

Iowa-trained psychologist Leon Yarrow was among the first maternal deprivation theorists to address the possible role of sensory deprivation. In 1951, Yarrow had abandoned a promising university career to join the U.S. Children's Bureau, where he pioneered longitudinal studies on adoption. His work served as the basis for a change in official governmental policy recommendations, favoring placing children for adoption as early as possible, thus minimizing time spent in institutions or foster homes. This interest in the care of orphaned children led Yarrow to the field of maternal deprivation.[10] In a 1961 review in the *Psychological Bulletin*, Yarrow delineated three different types of deprivation that occurred in the institutional setting: "sensory deprivation, social deprivation, and emotional deprivation." He relied on animal studies to argue that severe impairment could result from a child's early deprivation of sensory experience. Tying animal studies with observations on institutionalized children, Yarrow argued that even the most "extreme institutional environments" created sensory deprivation to a lesser degree than that described in animal studies. Still, he maintained, "developmental retardation is found, with the extent of retardation corresponding to the degree of sensory deprivation."[11]

For Yarrow, sensory deprivation was a major reason why institutional care of young infants should be avoided. Still, he criticized attempts to conflate maternal and sensory deprivation as well as efforts to isolate the components of maternal deprivation into variables of tactile, auditory, and visual deprivation, which he saw as reductionist endeavors that promoted overly simplified interpretations of experimental findings. It was likely, he added, "that not all aspects of the mother-child relationship can be meaningfully reduced to such simple variables."[12] Although Yarrow adopted much of the sensory deprivation language, he still assigned a specific role to the concept of mothering that could not be reduced completely to a form of stimulation.

Ainsworth had mixed feelings about these developments in the field. Although she did not comment directly on Yarrow's 1961 piece, she had previously commented on Yarrow's work in her letters to Bowlby. Describing

Yarrow's presentation at the American Psychological Association, she noted that he gave "considerable emphasis to the 'sensory deprivation' aspects of the institutional experience with . . . inadequate attention to the fact that it is in interpersonal interaction, especially with the mother, that the infant and young child experiences most of its 'sensory stimulation.'"[13] Ainsworth criticized in even stronger terms the responses of two leading figures in the field of educational psychology, Robert Sears and Joseph McVicker Hunt, whom she claimed

> welcomed the divorce of sensory stimulation from the child's relation-ship with his mother, as though it were personally satisfactory to think of a component that was free from the sentimental glorification of the child-mother relationship. It seems to me that this, which represents a fairly common viewpoint in American psychology, misses the whole point of trying to understand how it is that the child's relationship with his mother is so important for his development. When they find a variable such as sensory stimulation–deprivation they say "Aha! Here is something that is important that is impersonal and objective and for which the mother [as] such is not necessary." Instead it seems to me they should say "Here is a component of the child-mother relationship which we can identify, and which helps us understand why it is that, under usual conditions, maternal care is necessary for health develop-ment." . . . However, I got the impression that Yarrow, Sears and McV. Hunt felt that the sensory deprivation component quite accounted for all instances of impairment of intelligence attributable to separation. And certainly they quite ignore the clinical evidence pointing to the fact that repeated disruptions of the mother-child relationship may lead to very severe disturbances quite in the absence of institutionalization and "sensory deprivation." I found the whole thing quite discouraging.[14]

In a later letter to Yarrow, Ainsworth emphasized her preference for con-ceptualizing the role of maternal care in terms of the mother's relationship to the child rather than through biological or functional explanations. She was "uncomfortable," she explained, with Yarrow's "use of the term 'stimulation' when I would prefer the term 'interaction.'" Still, she conceded that "both the definitions you give of your maternal care variables and your discussion of your findings makes it clear that there is no substantial difference in our viewpoints." Both agreed that sensory deprivation research was an important component in the evaluation of maternal deprivation.[15]

While Yarrow and additional psychologists viewed maternal care within both biological and psychological frameworks, others focused solely on mothers' functional roles. In 1961, psychologist Lawrence Casler published "Maternal Deprivation: A Critical Review of the Literature," in which he effectively claimed that the detrimental effects attributed to "maternal deprivation" by Spitz, Bowlby, and others were in fact a result of reduced perceptual (or sensory) input. He suggested using "perceptual deprivation" rather than "the too-broad and yet too-specific term, 'maternal deprivation.'"[16] In particular, he argued that it was unlikely that maternal deprivation could occur in children under the age of six months, as a basic level of psychological matureness was necessary for the child to be able to respond to this form of deprivation."[17] Rather, the impediments to psychological and intellectual development that could be seen in institutionalized infants, he argued, resulted from a lack of sensory stimulation. His review extensively cited experiments from the field of sensory deprivation, both in human subjects and in animals.[18]

Ainsworth considered this review to be "quite horrible."[19] She wrote (but according to her records ultimately did not send) a detailed and highly critical letter to the editor of the monograph series that had published Casler's piece. Making her disapproval clear, she offered to prepare a monograph in response that would present the research in the field in a "more balanced and less distorted way than Casler presents it." This, she suggested, would be a reply to those who attempted to "translate maternal deprivation into sensory deprivation." Ainsworth also suggested examining "Yarrow's and Casler's urgings toward redefining 'maternal deprivation' as "sensory deprivation.'" She was willing to consider the importance of certain aspects of sensory deprivation within maternal deprivation, she wrote, but was steadfast in her rejection of attempts to redefine maternal deprivation as merely a form of sensory deprivation.[20]

Although she never prepared this critical review, in her 1962 article, "Deprivation of Maternal Care: Review of Findings and Controversy," published in a World Health Organization report on maternal deprivation, Ainsworth conceded that only in the early months of life was it "tenable" to argue that the child was suffering from "perceptual" deprivation rather than "maternal deprivation." At this age, she claimed, "'perceptual deprivation' seems equivalent to insufficiency of maternal care."[21] In this manner, Ainsworth turned the equation propounded by Casler and others on its head: Perceptual deprivation was in fact a form of maternal deprivation. In any case, theories of sensory deprivation clearly had pervaded the attachment theorist's view of maternal deprivation, and Ainsworth was now willing to explore the relevance of sensory deprivation theory to her study of mother-child interaction.

Although she did not perform her own research on sensory deprivation, Ainsworth gradually accepted this theory, participating in conferences on the topic, including a 1963 conference that also featured leading sensory deprivation researchers Donald Hebb and Austin Riesen.[22] In 1973, when she was asked to write a book on sensory deprivation (a request she ultimately declined because of time constraints), Ainsworth wrote that her interest in sensory deprivation stemmed from her work on the deprivation of maternal care. She had wanted to write a book on sensory deprivation, she attested, ever since she completed a review of the literature on maternal deprivation in 1962.[23]

Ainsworth was familiar with ongoing sensory deprivation research. She recommended Philip Solomon, a psychiatrist and leading researcher in the field of sensory deprivation, to an acquaintance who requested a reference for a psychiatrist. She was also on friendly terms with John Zubek, a Winnipeg sensory deprivation researcher, and in 1960 was invited to give a lecture at the University of Manitoba, where Zubek served as head of the psychology department.[24]

Ainsworth gradually became more open to examining sensory deprivation research and its relevance to her work on maternal deprivation. When a prospective student contacted her in 1965 to inquire about research in early parental deprivation, she suggested either programs carrying out research in sensory deprivation on animals, as at McGill University, or those focusing on cultural deprivation among African American children at the University of Chicago. Her home institution, Johns Hopkins, she explained, had only a small research program on social attachment, and it was not specifically focused on parental deprivation. The alternatives she suggested—sensory deprivation work on animals or cultural deprivation research—demonstrated the interrelations she saw among early childhood maternal or parental deprivation and laboratory research.[25]

In 1966, Ainsworth first corresponded with psychologist Joseph McVicker Hunt, whose work she had previously criticized for its overemphasis of sensory deprivation and inattention to the role of maternal care. In this letter, she highlighted the interconnections between her research on early infants and Hunt's research on the role of early experience in development of intelligence. Their work, she suggested, could "considerably overlap in viewpoint and interests." Her research on maternal deprivation had led her to the same

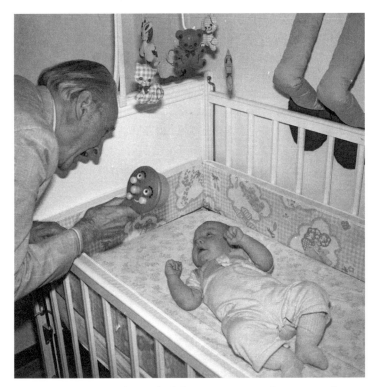

Joseph McVicker Hunt plays with a baby, 1977. Courtesy of University of
Illinois Archives, Urbana.

conclusions as Hunt reached: Early experience influenced later intelligence.
Not mincing words, she admitted that her previous work on the development
of intelligence following maternal deprivation was simply "wrong." Her new
approach, now saturated with biological terms, resembled Hunt's. "Under
circumstance of deprivation," she wrote, "the infant does not have the experience necessary to develop his sensory-motor schemata in the same way and
at the same rate that the average home-reared child has." Yet as the infant
matures, she wrote, "locomotion will develop"—a rather stilted way of saying that the toddler would soon be walking on his or her own. At that point,
the child could change his or her environment by moving from one place to
another, thereby obtaining the necessary stimulation for development. This
letter indicates the influence sensory deprivation theory and terminology had
on the development of Ainsworth's work, leading her to reevaluate her previous ideas and rethink them within a biologically oriented and stimulation-
based framework.[26]

Although it is quite possible that Ainsworth sought to highlight the similarities rather than the differences in approach when corresponding with an eminent biologically oriented psychologist such as Hunt, she told Bowlby of a similar change in her approach. Describing her planned participation in a symposium that she speculated would highlight biological views of development, she added, "In my new frame of mind, this does not dismay me."[27] She had unquestionably modified her early views of the relevance of sensory deprivation to understanding infant development, demonstrating her gradual acceptance of sensory deprivation at as an important theoretical approach.

René Spitz

Austrian-born émigré psychoanalyst René Spitz had a long-standing interest in the dangers of parental separation in early childhood. Well-known today for his early descriptions of the detrimental results of prolonged institutionalization or hospitalization of young infants, Spitz defined a new syndrome, anaclitic depression, that resulted when young infants were separated from their primary caregivers.[28] Unlike Ainsworth, Spitz's profound interest in the role of sensory deprivation was evident from his early writings. Spitz referred to perceptual and motor deprivation in his famed paper on "hospitalism" (a syndrome of prolonged institutionalization), which he published in 1945, long before sensory deprivation had permeated psychiatric discourse. In 1955, Spitz was invited to participate in the Regional Research Conference of the American Psychiatric Association, held in Montreal. He and Donald Hebb shared a session titled "Some After-Effects of Social Isolation in Animal and Man." Hebb delivered a talk on dogs reared in social isolation; Spitz spoke of the "somatic consequences of emotional starvation in infants."[29] In preparation for this talk and for his meeting with Hebb, Spitz read a number of articles by Hebb and his colleagues and had his assistant abstract and summarize Hebb's major publications.[30] Spitz opened his talk by stating that he had long followed Hebb's work, emphasizing that Hebb's experimental findings confirmed his own work. The idea that a psychoanalyst's research on mother-infant interactions could be empirically confirmed by experimental studies on human and animal subjects in laboratory conditions is not self-evident. Rather, it illustrates Spitz's acceptance of Hebb's experimental methodology and the close relations Spitz believed existed between maternal and sensory deprivation.[31] As a participant on the same panel as Hebb and particularly in his home city, Montreal, Spitz would certainly have felt compelled to highlight the importance of Hebb's work. Yet that Spitz would cite this work as evidence of the validity of his psychoanalytic research indicates a far greater acceptance of the relevance of sensory deprivation theory than would have been necessitated by standards of professional courtesy.

Indeed, Spitz saw many parallels between sensory deprivation research and his own work. Not addressing sensory deprivation was even a point of critique when he evaluated the works of his psychoanalyst colleagues.[32] In 1964, he claimed that "in the human infant, emotional deprivation without sensory and experimental deprivation is not possible," thus arguing that every case of maternal deprivation would necessarily have a component of sensory deprivation.[33] For Spitz, unlike Ainsworth, it was not a question of accepting sensory deprivation and its relevance for maternal deprivation; he viewed maternal and sensory deprivation as inherently linked.

Both Ainsworth and Spitz, who had pivotal roles in the development of seminal theories regarding the implications of maternal deprivation, saw the development of sensory deprivation theories as complementary to their approaches. Insights from sensory deprivation studies were readily incorporated into their thinking, fostering a broad interpretation of what the concept of childhood deprivation implied and what components were necessary for intellectual and psychological development. Maternal deprivation was seen as inextricably tied to sensory deprivation.

This merging of theories of maternal and sensory deprivation yielded interdisciplinary interpretations as researchers attempted to subsume the findings of sensory deprivation experiments into a psychoanalytic framework. Anthropologist Ashley Montagu suggested that "if we massage the skin in infancy, it may later be unnecessary for a physician to massage his psyche."[34] This viewpoint demonstrates the broad interpretations of sensory deprivation research and how it was viewed as salient to understanding a wide range of phenomena. Indeed, University of California at Los Angeles psychiatrist Stanley Cohen, basing his conclusions on a review of sensory deprivation experiments on animals, suggested adding to the Freudian stages of development a supplementary cutaneous stage in which all stimulus was transmitted through the skin. This suggestion, made in all seriousness, demonstrates that sensory deprivation research was seen as highly relevant for understanding psychoanalysis and was readily adopted and transferred into psychoanalytic discourses.[35]

The interface between theories of sensory and maternal deprivation gave rise to practical interventions. Casler, who saw maternal deprivation as simply one case of sensory deprivation, devised three experimental interventions examining the role of specific forms of stimulation.[36] In a study examining the effects of extra tactile stimulation on institutionalized infants, the impersonal language Casler employed is striking: "Two young women, designated hereafter as 'handlers,'" he explained, "were hired to administer the tactile stimulation."[37] Designed as a case-control intervention, the "handlers" would provide the children in the case group with two ten-minute periods of "additional tactile stimulation" while saying "Hello, Baby" once every sixty seconds. The control group received only the greeting, without the tactile stimulation. This greeting was delivered "in a neutral tone and without smiling" to "minimize the possibility that the subject would respond to 'affection' rather than to skin contact."[38] The results indicated, according to Casler, that the babies who received extra stimulation functioned at a higher level and scored higher on tests evaluating their language development and their personality characteristics.[39] As a result of his findings, Casler argued that if satisfactory sensory stimulation could be provided in institutions, "there is reason to ask whether mother love remains a variable of importance in infant development."[40] Thus the replacement of the concept of maternal deprivation by sensory deprivation led to the development of specific interventions, described in this case as "extra handling" of infants.

The Debate over Day Care—
Sensory or Maternal Deprivation?

Within a few years, theories of sensory deprivation supplemented and even replaced those of maternal deprivation. The interface between these two theories gained particular significance in the debate over child day care throughout the 1960s. Theories of deprivation, child development theories, public policy, and American politics all converged in the contentious discussion of child care arrangements.[41] With the ever-increasing rise in women's employment, suitable child care became a necessity. Experts in child development warned of the substandard conditions available to some children whose mothers worked and who were left with older siblings or neighbors or in understaffed and unqualified group homes. During World War II, when women were employed in war-related industries, descriptions of children left in parked cars while their mothers worked long hours in factories aroused public concern. In 1942, under the Lanham Act, the government allocated funds for the care of children whose mothers were engaged in wartime industries. Matching state funds, federal money supported local child care centers, which opened in forty-seven states. Under severe time and budgetary constraints, most centers were of questionable educational quality, but they at least answered the needs of working mothers. Yet the end of the war led to the abrupt end of federal funding for child care, and few facilities subsequently were available for infants and toddlers.[42]

New trends in child development theory led experts to underscore the psychological and intellectual benefits of early child educational programs. Furthermore, descriptions of the highly effective Soviet educational system, which began with very young children and molded productive and precocious schoolchildren, led Cold War American child development experts to wonder whether waiting to begin formal education with kindergarten placed Americans at an educational disadvantage.[43]

Yet alongside this surge of interest in day care, the threat of "maternal deprivation" and animosity toward maternal employment still dampened interest in early child education. Child care scholar Sonya Michel has argued that the most vehement opposition to both maternal employment and the establishment of day care facilities was voiced by psychologists.[44] The research by Bowlby, Spitz, and others on the dangers of maternal deprivation had in fact examined the detrimental effect of prolonged separation from the mother combined with institutionalization, often in conditions that provided very little beyond food and shelter. Yet their findings were seen as applicable to all forms of maternal separation, regardless of length or alternative caring arrangements provided. Many observers viewed maternal deprivation as a real threat even in the case of short and reversible separations between children and their mothers. These psychological theories of maternal deprivation were used to encourage young mothers to stay at home.[45]

Most child development experts envisioned a mother caring for her young children in her own home as the ideal situation and consequently saw maternal employment as a sign of pathology, either sociocultural (poverty required the mother to work) or psychological (for middle-class mothers). Women who worked were seen as having psychological difficulties in accepting their natural social role. Psychologically compelled to compete with their male counterparts—suffering from "penis envy" or sublimating their personal frustrations—working mothers were subjected to a variety of unflattering interpretations.[46] Mental health experts put much effort into elucidating those personality characteristics that led mothers to choose to work, a choice that clearly was not seen as self-explanatory.[47] As a result, day care was seen as a "problem service," provided for children of working mothers in low-income homes or prescribed by social workers for children from inadequate homes. Such children were removed from their homes for certain hours each day, regardless of their mothers' employment status.[48]

The question of deprivation played a pivotal role in the public and professional debate on the merits of day care and the different sectors for whom it would be beneficial. On the one hand, day care programs were designed to provide children from low-income families with the stimulation they lacked in their impoverished home environments. On the other hand, maternal deprivation theorists expressed their worries about separating children from their mothers. These perceptions were closely tied to race and class. Low-income and minority children were seen to benefit from the separation from their mothers and the placement in day care programs, while middle-class children were seen to be at risk for maternal deprivation. Sensory deprivation theories were also invoked in the debate over cultural deprivation and remedial education, as will be seen in the following chapter.

By the early 1960s, as women rallied for equal rights and opportunities, middle-class women were touting child care arrangements as a means to ensure professional advancement. Faced with the inevitability of increasingly large numbers of children requiring care outside of their homes as American society seemed poised on the brink of social change, child development experts altered their perceptions of child care to fit the times. These experts gradually attempted to reframe day care programs no longer as solely custodial solutions but instead as conferring developmental benefits. Looking back, child psychologist Bettye Caldwell and pediatrician Julius Richmond recalled that "during the late 1950s and early 1960s a sure path to ostracism in the field of early childhood education was to emphasize attendance at nursery school as an influence on intellectual development."[49] By the mid-1960s, however, early childhood education was widely accepted as having significant developmental and psychological benefits. These benefits, however, were seen to be mainly applicable to low-income and minority children. Child care historian Elly Singer has claimed that while the benefit in terms of cognitive development was emphasized in evaluations of child care programs for children from low-income families, studies of child care for middle-class children focused on the negative emotional effects of separation from their mothers.[50] This discrepancy can be understood through the differential interpretations of sensory and maternal deprivation according to class and race. In an article published in a 1963 World Health Organization review of child care centers,

Julius Richmond, who later became the director of Head Start and served as the U.S. surgeon general, provided a historical overview of how sensory deprivation research had led to a reevaluation and reframing of maternal deprivation theory and argued that through careful design, maternal deprivation could be avoided when providing day care for young children.[51] By the middle of the decade, however, the emphasis changed from how to avoid the deprivation that might be caused by day care to how day care could counter the deprivation that afflicted children from minority and low-income homes.

One of the earliest remedial interventions was designed by Caldwell and Richmond, both of whom were at the State University of New York in Syracuse at the time. This early childhood enrichment program, which opened its doors in 1964, was designed "to develop powers of sensory and perceptual discrimination, an orientation toward activity, and the feeling of mastery and personal accomplishment." Focusing on children from low-income homes, the program later served as the model for Head Start.[52] In their eight-page description of their proposed program, the words "deprived" and "deprivation" appear thirteen times, referring to sensory deprivation, cultural deprivation, and maternal deprivation. The program targeted children from low-income homes with working mothers and described those children as deprived. There was no mention of the children's ethnic background. The authors attempted to distinguish between the deprivations that already afflicted the children (sensory deprivation, environmental impoverishment) and maternal deprivation, which, they contended, was not an inevitable result of the intervention. "The basic hypothesis to be tested," Caldwell and Richmond explained, was "that an appropriate environment can be programmed which will offset any developmental detriment associated with maternal separation and possibly add a degree of environmental enrichment frequently not available in families of limited social, economic, and cultural resource."[53] Thus, the authors in fact proposed that the benefits of environmental enrichments that would compensate for deprived homes would outweigh the potential risk of separating children from their mothers.

Describing the early results of the Syracuse Children's Center, Caldwell and Richmond argued that "inadequate sensory input during the early years is strongly implicated as one of the factors involved in the early learning deficit so often shown by the child who grows up in an environment of poverty." Accordingly, efforts were made "to provide variety in intensities of sensory input, color, shape, texture, sound patterns, etc." Even the necessity of maintaining order within the child care center was ascribed to sensory theory:

"The maintenance of order is an essential aspect of the sensory environment and is crucial to help the child distinguish figure from background, particularly for the child whose home environment may be somewhat crowded or even chaotic."[54] The need for an orderly environment as a value in itself apparently was not sufficiently self-evident, and the authors relied instead on deprivation theory to highlight its importance. Caldwell and her student collaborators argued in a later article that "we *have* offered environmental enrichment, and we *have* shown that it is possible to do this without producing the classical picture of maternal deprivation."[55] This polarization of sensory deprivation (the target of the intervention) and maternal deprivation (not an inevitable side effect of the separation) is characteristic of descriptions of interventions designed for children from low-income families during this era.

Caldwell elsewhere argued that the "optimal environment" for young infants would be in their own homes, "in the context of a warm, continuous emotional relationship with his own mother under conditions of varied sensory input." Yet not all mothers, Caldwell continued, were capable of providing the care and stimulation young infants needed. Lamenting the absence of a "literacy test for motherhood," she cited researchers who had found evidence of inadequate parenting abilities among low-income mothers. Early intervention programs provided what she described as the "professionalization of the mother-substitute" role. By providing a surrogate mother alongside adequate stimulation, the early intervention program headed by Richmond and Caldwell would counter sensory deprivation without leading to maternal deprivation.[56]

In a special 1965 issue of the journal *Child Welfare* devoted to the question of day care, a program director at a child day care facility in New York argued that the separation of children from their mothers was not necessarily harmful. He went so far as to venture that perhaps "day care can offer something valuable to children *because* they are separated from their parents?"[57] Another article in the same issue described a "day care service that is perceived and operated as a social service for parents and children of low socioeconomic status." This service was provided to children "whose family situations do not contribute to their best interests." The article made no reference to maternal deprivation but included detailed descriptions of the interventions designed to offset cultural deprivation, including linguistic learning, development of perception, conceptualization, and self-identification.[58] Thus, the separation itself from the home and the low-income working mother was seen as therapeutic rather than pathogenic. Deprivation was depicted as the target of the intervention rather than an unwanted outcome of the separation of children from their mothers. Although the discussion of maternal separation made no specific mention of race, the article was based on the work at Seven Hills Neighborhood Houses, an inner-city housing agency that served mainly African Americans and migrants from the Appalachian area.[59]

Many educators at this time held that children from different socioeconomic backgrounds had different needs. This distinction was made abundantly clear in an article by Eleanor Hosley, executive director of the Cleveland Day Nursery Association, a nonprofit early child care association that had been established in 1882. Hosley described the different groups of children that could be observed at the day care centers. Children of working mothers "must spend" most of their waking hours in a day care center and thus "desperately need the enriching educational experiences that might be expected to be provided by their mother could she be with them." Thus, the day care center would provide compensation for the time that children of working mothers spent away from them. In contrast, the child "who lives in a city slum with crowds of people who have neither the time nor the knowledge to devote to his special needs also requires an enriched background, whether or not his mother has employment." Finally, children of the rich "whose parents are constantly on the go" also required such attention, and "therefore the process of meeting the needs of the culturally deprived preschool child from low-income areas involves the same basic essentials as the education of the 3- and 4-year-olds of more privileged background."[60] Although the author attested to the similarity of the needs of children from different socioeconomic strata, the subtext of her description was that some children needed compensation for being separated from their parents, while others should be separated from their parents *as* a form of therapeutic intervention. There was no mention of race; furthermore, when Hosley later mentioned race in the article, she did so to draw attention to the devastating effects of discrimination on children's self-esteem.[61] Yet the description of the "slum" children living in poverty in inner-city Cleveland, alongside the fact that the day care program for low-income children served a classroom that was 90 percent African American, left little room for doubt about the subtext.[62] For Hosley, removing children of color from their inadequate home environments was therapeutic in itself, regardless of whether or not their mothers were employed.

These comparisons between the needs of low-income and middle-class children appeared in many publications on early child care. Menninger Clinic psychologist Lois Murphy described middle-class children as often being "over-mothered and overstimulated," while mothers of deprived children cannot "provide the stimulation that most middle-class children receive. . . . [C]onversation may be squelched and curiosity discouraged." The day care consultant's role was to evaluate the child's background and determine the form of intervention needed for the individual child.[63]

As late as 1975, by which time early child care had gained widespread acceptability and no longer was recommended solely for children of low-income families, an article in the *American Journal of Orthopsychiatry* was wary of the possible adverse effects of day care on middle-class children. The author argued that just because children from impoverished environments were not adversely affected by full-time day care did not mean that the same held true for children "from more stimulating middle-class homes" since the "nature of the mother-child relationship and the development of competence in infancy is known to differ across socioeconomic levels."[64] This distinction between the different needs of children of different socioeconomic levels and the role accorded to day care for each group—therapeutic for low-income families, depriving for the middle class—persisted and had a lasting influence on the development of child care programs.

Mothers as the Mediators of Deprivation

While some early child care experts attempted to distinguish between maternal deprivation, a phenomenon used nearly exclusively to describe middle-class children separated from their mothers, and sensory deprivation, which afflicted lower-class children who remained at home with their mothers, others attempted to conflate the two concepts. Some psychologists sought to depict the mother as the mediator of all forms of deprivation, maternal and sensory. Early childhood educators David Weikart and Dolores Lambie created the Ypsilanti Home Teaching Project, which involved sending teachers "into the homes of disadvantaged families to provide a training program for the mother and a tutoring program for the preschool child." Approximately 75 percent of the participating families were white. The researchers examined the different characteristics of the mothers participating in the program, who were rated by the participating teachers by what the authors described as a "general 'good-bad' dimension." The authors concluded that "it is not social-economic status that determines cognitive deprivation but lack of warmth and verbal communication by the mother."[65] In the face of life's adverse circumstances, the mother was credited for providing an adequate environment. Yet in cases when the creation of such an adequate environment was not feasible as a consequence of poverty, illness, insufficient opportunities, and lack of support, the mother was at fault. A "good" mother would have been able to create the necessary surroundings for the child's optimal development. Similarly, Lois Murphy propounded a "concept of vulnerability" that took into account both socioeconomic status and "adequacy" of mothering. According to her classification, "high risk mothers" were those who suffered from "sensory defects, deficiencies of strength, energy, or physical resources, as well as apathy, depression, extreme passivity, excessive lability, and marked irritability or hostility." These inadequate mothers were depicted as suffering from deficiencies of every kind, from sensory deficits to deficits of psychological and physiological abilities. In this case, not only were children from low-income homes viewed as deprived but their mothers too were conceptualized through a framework highlighting their lacks and deficiencies.[66]

Many psychologists accorded mothers a central role in the prevention of deprivation. Ainsworth and her former student Silvia Bell depicted mothers as the mediators of deprivation or of adequate development. While Ainsworth and Bell conceded that the home conditions associated with "socioeconomic deprivation" detrimentally affected cognitive development, such conditions were seen as secondary to adequate mothering: A "harmonious infant-mother relationship can act as a buffer protecting a child from their detrimental effect, and, in fact is the single most important factor alleviating socioeconomic disadvantage."[67]

At some level, this approach empowered low-income mothers, who were seen as potentially competent and responsible for the fate of their children; however, it also reinterpreted the results of the detrimental effects of poverty and lack of opportunities as consequences of maternal behavior. Thus, the effects of poverty were transposed into a psychological discourse, shifting the responsibility from society or the government to the individual mother. Subsequent interventions focused not on ameliorating the dismal living conditions of these impoverished families, creating job opportunities, and providing governmental assistance but rather on educating mothers to act more effectively as buffers against the influence of adverse life circumstances.

The practical implications of this approach were the components of in-home interventions designed to train mothers to better stimulate their children. Such programs sent educators into the homes of low-income families, teaching deprived mothers to mitigate the effects of deprivation on their children.[68]

Some child development researchers compared the educational and developmental role of the mother to that of the day care teacher. Middle-class mothers were described as spontaneously acting like teachers in child-centered nursery schools, turning their homes into learning environments. Conversely, other researchers argued that an "ideal day care program" provided child rearing equivalent to that provided by active, middle-class mothers.[69] This was sometimes viewed as a form of compensation for inadequate mothering. Psychologist Lois Murphy wrote that the "kind of things a 'good' mother does with a year-old baby may be helpful for these children [from "deprived" backgrounds] at a much older age."[70] Having been deprived of a good mother in infancy, these children could enjoy the substitute maternal care provided by nursery school teachers.

Implicitly or sometimes quite openly, these child development experts claimed that preschool offered no developmental benefits to middle-class children beyond providing custodial solutions when the mother was unavailable to care for her children. In contrast, removing lower-class children from their impoverished surroundings and placing them in day care facilities could be seen as the equivalent to placing such children with the middle-class mothers they so lacked and thus instilling in them the values and care they were deprived of at home.[71] Hence, while emphasizing the role of early child care in promoting intellectual development was no longer "a sure path to ostracism," its benefits were mainly viewed as applying to children from low-income homes.[72] Middle-class children still risked the detrimental effects of separation from their mothers, who remained the ultimate ideal source of education and stimulation.

Deprivation and Policymaking: Income Maintenance Programs

Government committees evaluating child care programs in the mid- and late 1960s sought the opinions of experts in the field of maternal deprivation and child development. In 1968, Lyndon Baines Johnson appointed the President's Commission on Income Maintenance Programs. Chaired by business leader Ben Heineman, the commission was designed to evaluate possible welfare reform strategies.[73] The initial prospect of an income maintenance program received much support on the political left, whose members did not believe, as conservative critics suggested, that a guaranteed income was incompatible with the ideal of individual advancement through hard work and education. Rather, income maintenance proponents touted such a program as a way to supplement low wages and thereby assist low-paid workers in rising from poverty. The commission set out to examine how income maintenance could be compatible both with encouraging individuals to work and with providing a safety net for the working poor. One of the questions the commission addressed was who would be required to work to be eligible for government benefits. Requiring mothers of young children to seek employment would clearly necessitate an overreaching reform of day care services. Thus, Dr. Iris Rotberg, a specialist in education policy and commission staff member, surveyed leading psychologists, including Ainsworth, for their opinion on the widespread implementation of early day care programs.[74] Ainsworth replied in detail, distinguishing between day care programs designed to take care of children of working mothers and those designed to "provide stimulation to intellectual development to infants and young children in disadvantaged segments of the population." She provided a critical overview of the current approach to early child care, which was designed "to supplement family care and to provide the stimulation the child lacks and home," arguing that "many experts on pre-school education fear that this kind of emphasis might very well do damage through a lop-sided emphasis on cognitive development— over-stimulation, etc." As opposed to this "new-fangled" approach to day care, which emphasized sensory stimulation, Ainsworth described the "more old-fashioned notion of day care," which was to "simply to look after the children of working mothers." In this case, Ainsworth warned, it was necessary to attempt to "minimize the effects of deprivation (whether this is considered to be 'maternal deprivation' or deprivation of stimulation)," which could be analogized to the experience of infants in long-term residential facilities, by means of adequate staffing and individual attention. Distinguishing between the two different purposes of day care, Ainsworth added that to her knowledge, "no one was bold enough to propose removing children from adequate homes in order to give them whatever advantages day care of an enlightened kind might have."[75]

Thus Ainsworth distinguished between remedial day care programs, which were potentially useful for children from deprived homes regardless of maternal employment, and programs targeting nondeprived children of working mothers, which should use adequate staffing to avoid maternal deprivation. Rotberg confided in Ainsworth that she suspected "that in the real world any extensive or broad based day care system could not be staffed with perceptive, stable and interested caretakers" such as those provided in "model" programs. After requesting input from a number of leading psychologists and child development experts, Rotberg ultimately recommended that the criterion of employment be excluded when determining the eligibility of mothers of young children for public assistance, a recommendation adopted by the Income Maintenance Commission.[76] Requiring women to work and providing the day care facilities to enable them to do so were not steps the commission was willing to condone. The report stated that stipulating the provision of day care on maternal employment or training was "costly, narrowly conceived, and coercive."[77]

Following the distinction Ainsworth had suggested, the report compared "purely custodial care" with childhood enrichment, reaching the same conclusion Rotberg had articulated in her letter to Ainsworth. Developing a real enrichment program with a satisfactory adult-to-child ratio would be too great a challenge. The report concluded that if day care was regarded as an "important child development opportunity," it should be offered universally as an extension of public education and not as a method to "coerce" the "poor mother to work regardless of their skills, abilities and desires."[78]

The commission recommended the creation of a national income supplement program. It would provide a base minimum income, which would be reduced by fifty cents for each dollar of income from other sources, thus providing an incentive for participants to continue working.[79] The commission did not complete its evaluation until 1969, and the new president, Richard Nixon, partially adopted its recommendations in the Family Assistance Plan (FAP). The FAP, announced in 1969, was designed to guarantee the indigent a fixed income level and would require work from all but mothers of small children. Responding to growing dissatisfaction with the Aid to Families with Dependent Children Act, which provided benefits to single mothers, it is ironic that Nixon ultimately proposed a welfare reform that promised a guaranteed income to all. Particularly at a time when the public was deeply dissatisfied with antipoverty measures, which were often seen as perpetuating dependency and being "abused" by African Americans, Nixon's FAP might seem surprising. Yet as Marisa Chappell has argued, this plan in fact embodied a deeply conservative view of the family, designed to strengthen the position of the male breadwinner by rewarding work rather than penalizing it through reduced benefits and to reduce the incentive for single mothers to work.[80] Severely criticized by both liberals and conservatives, the bill was allowed to disappear quietly in 1972, avoiding controversy in an election year.[81] Work requirement for welfare eligibility did not resurface for more than four decades, until the passage of President Bill Clinton's over-arching welfare reform, the Personal Responsibility and Work Opportunity Reconciliation Act, which contained strict work requirements, including for mothers of young children.[82]

Universal Day Care—Why Not?

In 1971, President Nixon vetoed the Economic Opportunity Amendments, which were designed to serve as an extension of the Economic Opportunity Act of 1964 and included the establishment of a comprehensive child de-velopment program that would have served as the legal basis for providing universal day care.[83] Nixon criticized the entire package but found the Child Development Act "the most deeply flawed provision of this legislation," con-demning its "fiscal irresponsibility, administrative unworkability, and family-weakening implications." Under pressure from conservative politicians and activists, Nixon instead approved extensive tax deductions for child care expenses, demonstrating what has been termed a "hidden welfare" policy.[84]

This policy of direct provision only for the neediest people while pro-viding tax benefits for the middle class has been revised numerous times but nevertheless still characterizes the current state of U.S. funding for child care. Currently, while most mothers of young children of preschool age are employed, the nation has no universal state-sponsored system of preschool child care such as exists in Australia, France, Japan, or the Scandinavian coun-tries.[85] Children from low-income families are eligible for federally subsi-dized care, while middle- and upper-class families benefit from indirect sup-port in the form of tax rebates and deductions.[86] At first look, this differential system might seem surprising. Since both child development experts and politicians held that early child care was beneficial, rallying behind programs such as Head Start, it would seem logical that policymakers would argue that such care should be available to all. Yet, as David Rothman has shown, many federal programs developed in the 1960s and early 1970s that might have been expected to raise awareness to the necessity of universal access to certain services in fact achieved the opposite effect.[87] Rather than ques-tioning the wisdom of minimizing government involvement and maximizing individual choice and the free market, certain exceptions further crystallized the reliance on these same principles. For example, the decision to provide funding for all dialysis patients by federal law in 1972 did not promote more awareness of other catastrophic illnesses in which universal health coverage might be warranted.[88] Similarly, the acceptance that early child care could be beneficial for intellectual and psychological development did not lead to the conclusion that it should be available to all. Class and race-specific interpretations of deprivation helped present early child care as an exception to the rule of minimal government intervention and free-market exchange of services but did not lead people to question whether these principles should be in play in the debate over early education.

The 1971 Child Development Act had originated from two separate bills developed by Senator Walter Mondale, a Minnesota Democrat, and Representative John Brademas, a Democrat from Indiana. As the name implies, the bill highlighted the developmental benefits afforded by early education, modeling itself after the perceived success of Project Head Start. The Mondale-Brademas proposal was unique in that it depicted early child care as providing developmental benefits rather than as solely a custodial solution. Accordingly, it sought to confer this developmental benefit universally, not only to children from low-income homes. The bill would have provided federally subsidized child care to middle-class families on the basis of a sliding-scale fee system. At first, this proposal garnered bipartisan support, as liberal-leaning Senate Republicans such as New York's Jacob Javits and Pennsylvania's Richard Schweiker joined to cosponsor the bill. Furthermore, the bill's supporters depicted it as complementing the Nixon-backed FAP, providing the infrastructure of quality child care necessary to enable welfare reform that encouraged maternal employment. The bill eventually gained cosponsorship from 120 House members, approximately a third of them Republicans. Yet negotiations to accommodate the demands of community leaders and feminist activists invested in a community-action structure that would maximize local governance and minimize federal oversight led to the insertion of community-action principles in the bill. Much of the political wrangling centered on the level at which programs would receive direct federal support: The government preferred to award funds to states and large institutions, while local activists pushed to allow grants to small grassroots groups. The proposal originally provided funding primarily at the state level but allowed cities with populations above five hundred thousand to apply for autonomous child care systems; community activists, however, negotiated the threshold downward to five thousand, effectively bypassing state involvement and closely aligning the plan with the Great Society's community action programs. Conservatives as well as many liberals worried that these changes would prove structurally unwieldy. Furthermore, as the FAP fell out of favor among conservative politicians, conservative support waned for a bill depicted as FAP's auxiliary child care program.[89] The community action aspect of the bill alienated Republican supporters, who viewed these principles as radical and reeking of socialism. Particularly in light of the urban race riots of the mid- and late 1960s, community action programs had become anathema to conservative politicians, who accused activists of inciting violence and disorder. Thus, the rejection of the Child Development Act also formed part of the backlash against Johnson's Great Society programs and the principle of "maximum feasible participation."[90]

In an already contentious political atmosphere, including a debate over Nixon's renewed diplomatic relations with China, which aroused conservative wrath, the Child Development Act was highly controversial. As the bill's Republican supporters distanced themselves from the final proposal, Nixon faced an extremely vocal opposition. An orchestrated letter-writing campaign warned Nixon against destroying the American family.[91] Conservative pundits portrayed this bill as an attempt to "Sovietize" American society—and in particular, vulnerable children—by providing collective group care and weakening American family values.[92] While the right wing fought against the bill, activists who highlighted its community action aspect led more mainstream groups to lose interest in the support. Although the National Organization of Women had originally been a staunch supporter of universal day care as a means to promote mothers' rights, this influential group was marginalized in a debate that became transformed into a power struggle between two extremes.[93]

Nixon's veto of the Child Development Act after his previous public support for more accessible child care clearly reflected the political pressures exerted on the president as well as his personal preferences and biases. Child care was "ok for social workers," he stated bluntly in private meetings, but constituted "bad politics."[94] When it became clear that the FAP proposal was doomed to fail, Nixon lost interest in child care reform. He had no desire to provide middle-class children with what was touted as a developmental benefit: His primary interest had been in providing a custodial solution to encourage the employment of low-income mothers.[95] Never an outspoken advocate of women's rights, Nixon's views of day care were similar to those he held on abortion: Both should be available to poor women in dire straits

but should not be seen as a universal right designed to promote women's individual freedom.[96]

Although liberal backers of Project Head Start had initially worried that the Republican president would erode the program's political backing, Nixon had reaffirmed his belief in compensatory education as a means by which to target perceived deprivation. In a 1969 message to Congress on the anti-poverty programs, Nixon argued that "so crucial is the matter of early growth that we must make a national commitment to providing all American children an opportunity for healthful and stimulating development during the first five years of life." This commitment, according to Nixon, was exemplified in his controversial decision to move Project Head Start from the Office of Economic Opportunity to the Department of Health, Education, and Welfare.[97] Many child development experts criticized this decision, as the program's supporters feared that the move would "emasculate the concept of comprehensive child development programs," changing the focus from a comprehensive outlook on the child's home and community to a narrow view of education.[98] Nixon's wording clearly echoed deprivation-based approaches, as he referred to the necessity of stimulation during childhood and added that "many of the problems of poverty are traceable directly to early childhood experience," a view shared by many early educators and mental health professionals.[99]

Nixon made specific reference to this earlier commitment in his 1971 veto, emphasizing that he was not shirking his responsibility to provide early childhood education by rejecting the proposal for universal child care. The Child Development Act, he argued, went "far beyond what this administration envisioned." Nixon accepted the need to provide day care "to enable mothers, particularly those at the lowest income levels, to take full-time jobs." Furthermore, "the protection of children from actual suffering and deprivation," he argued, was an "imperative." These needs, however, were already seen as sufficiently addressed by Project Head Start, the Social Security Act, and child health and preventive care through Medicaid. For nondeprived children, however, the proposed bill had dangerous implications, diminishing "both parental authority and parental involvement with children" and "altering the family relationship" by working against efforts to bring "the family together." Thus, while day care provided an environment that enhanced growth and development and was presented as a positive service with many health and cognitive benefits, it offered these benefits only for lower-class children. Nixon held the risks of diminishing familial authority, separating children from parents, and reconfiguring the family structure as too great for children from middle-class families. When child care arrangements for middle-class children were necessary, Nixon believed, the federal government should play only a limited part: The "Federal Government's role wherever possible should be one of assisting parents to purchase needed day care services in the private, open market, with Federal involvement in direct provision of such services kept to an absolute minimum." This limited role contrasted starkly to the federal involvement deemed necessary for children eligible for Head Start— children from culturally and ethnically diverse and low-income backgrounds. For them, federal involvement was seen as beneficial.[100]

Middle-class mothers were perceived as choosing to take on employment and consequently were expected to make private arrangements for child care.[101] In contrast, children from low-income families were held to have an acute need for early childhood education, a need that the president believed the federal government had both an obligation and a clear incentive to fulfill. For middle-class children, however, early day care was seen to be risky, an unacceptable meddling in normative family life. Nixon's dual approach to day care—positive for the deprived levels of society but dangerous and depriving for the middle class—demonstrates the tension between theories of maternal and sensory deprivation. Concerned citizens, child development experts, politicians, and even the president believed that compensatory day care programs were necessary for children from low-income or "deprived" homes. Yet in the case of an adequate home, day care centers were seen as serving at best a custodial function and as potentially harmful, separating children from adequate mothers.

Conclusion

By the early 1960s, a decade after the term "maternal deprivation" was first coined, authors examining maternal deprivation dedicated a substantial proportion of their publications to the interrelations between sensory and maternal deprivation. Yet this discussion did not remain solely theoretical. The tension between these two concepts shaped the discourse over day care in the United States. Although it would be a stretch to claim that the entire debate over day care can be reduced to these two concepts, their selective application to families of differing socioeconomic strata provides a useful starting point for a historical understanding of America's lack of a coherent approach to child care.

Furthermore, this examination of the debate over day care exemplifies the connections between the expert discourse of child development professionals and public policy. While policymakers were certainly influenced by research carried out by child development experts, prevailing stereotypes of both lower-class and middle-class mothers as well as researchers' personal views on how mothers should raise their children influenced presuppositions and research hypotheses. Theories of sensory deprivation (and later cultural deprivation) were invoked in derogatory descriptions of low-income mothers and were put to use in advocating selective separation of children from their inadequate mothers to provide necessary components that were seen to be missing. Similarly, maternal deprivation theories were invoked to sway young middle-class mothers to stay at home with their children, instilling a dread of separation from the child for fear of creating irreversible deficiencies. Yet in both cases, the focus was on what children lacked rather than on their strengths, capabilities, or singularities, demonstrating how deeply ingrained the deprivation model had become.

CHAPTER TWO

Cultural Deprivation?

Race, Deprivation, and the Nature-Nurture Debate

DURING THE 1960S, cultural deprivation was the conceptual axis by which poverty and its long-term detrimental effects were viewed. The theory of cultural deprivation considered poverty not simply an economic condition but rather a distinct sociocultural pathology that caused academic and even intellectual disadvantage and social disability. Even worse, it created an additional generation of culturally deprived individuals, thus perpetuating the cycle of poverty.[1] Throughout the decade, the concept of cultural deprivation shaped how scientists, clinicians, and government officials perceived the abilities, needs, and home environments of children from families of differing socioeconomic statuses.

Cultural deprivation was closely tied to the theory of a culture of poverty, first articulated by University of Illinois anthropologist Oscar Lewis. Deeply committed to the study of poverty and inequality, Lewis spent extended periods carrying out ethnographic studies of impoverished families in Latin America. In 1959, he published *Five Families: Mexican Case Studies in the Culture of Poverty*, based on in-depth interviews and life stories.[2] Lewis coined the term "culture of poverty" to refer to the destructive behaviors and values he believed rendered the poor dependent and passive, unable to break the cycle of poverty in which they were enmeshed. This culture of poverty, Lewis postulated, transcended "regional, rural-urban and even national" boundaries; the poor had a culture of their own. Anticipating later uses of his theory, Lewis described "remarkable similarities" in numerous areas, including family structure and dynamics, between the poor families he had interviewed in Mexico and "lower-class Negroes" in the United States.[3] In 1961, Lewis published a second book based on taped interviews he had carried out with members of the Sanchez family, one of the original five families he had interviewed.[4] The book was read with much interest by Michael Harrington, a socialist activist and poverty scholar who in 1962 published

The Other America: Poverty in the United States. This book owed an intellectual debt to Lewis's work, as Harrington used the culture of poverty thesis to describe the poor in the United States.[5] Harrington's book, which sold seventy thousand copies in its first year, has been credited for mobilizing the American public to address the problem of poverty and for providing an important impetus for President John F. Kennedy and his successor, Lyndon Baines Johnson, to take an interest in antipoverty action.[6]

The cultural deprivation theory, popularized in the early 1960s, resembled the culture of poverty approach in that both theories were used to describe a distinct culture that was seen to have developed among low-income and mainly minority populations.[7] While the idea of cultural deprivation can in many ways be seen as a development of the culture of poverty approach and some scholars of poverty have used the terms interchangeably, I believe that the cultural deprivation theory was distinctive in its reliance on theories of deprivation popular at the time. In this chapter, I first outline the contested trajectory of the term "cultural deprivation" and then examine how research on this concept was derived from the established fields of sensory, maternal, and nutritional deprivation. No experiential evidence backed the theory of cultural deprivation; researchers cited data from studies examining other forms of deprivation. Thus, cultural deprivation was based on a racially and socioeconomically distinct interpretation of maternal and sensory deprivation. Theories of deprivation played an important role in the debate over language ability and acquisition among African American children and in explanations of the achievement gap in scholastic tests designed to measure intelligence. I examine the role of different theories of deprivation in the debates over the education of "culturally deprived" children before discussing the debate concerning psychologist Arthur Jensen's critique of compensatory education, in which he first articulated his hereditarian approach to intelligence.

Cultural Deprivation

The term "cultural deprivation" was ill defined and often contested. In social psychologist and antipoverty activist Frank Riessman's 1962 book, *The Culturally Deprived Child*, which contains one of the earliest uses of the term, the author stated in a footnote that he used the terms "culturally deprived," "educationally deprived," "deprived," "underprivileged," "disadvantaged," "lower-class," and "lower socioeconomic group" interchangeably through-out the book.[8]

The group to whom the term was applied was also undefined and contro-versial. One author wrote that "it is clear that almost 100 percent of the poor are culturally deprived," while other researchers stated that cultural depriva-tion was a "poor concept" as the "children encountered on their own grounds are not empty vessels, waiting to be filled with middle-class culture."[9] Yet despite the vagueness of the term and the controversy it elicited, the concept of cultural deprivation prevailed in 1960s medical, educational, and political discourse.

The architects of early antipoverty measures in the Kennedy and John-son administrations tried to avoid the depiction of their work as an African American or civil rights issue, focusing instead on rural pockets of poverty, particularly in Appalachia. Yet the success of this effort at avoiding questions of race proved short-lived.[10] By the mid-1960s, the "culturally deprived" had been transformed into a near euphemism for the urban, poor black commu-nity.[11] The racial overtones of the cultural deprivation theory raised many eyebrows, and even in its heyday in the early and mid-1960s, the theory was not without its critics. Many of those critics were African American scholars who rejected a theory that devalued black culture and family life.

Yet views on cultural deprivation were not divided strictly according to race. Some African American scholars viewed the cultural deprivation theory as an important contribution to understanding barriers to scholastic achieve-ment in their community. University of Chicago social anthropologist Allison Davis was active in developing the cultural deprivation approach; educator and Head Start researcher William Brazziel also embraced a compensatory approach designed to meet deprivations, although recommending sensitiv-ity in using the term "cultural deprivation."[12] In contrast, leading African American psychologist Kenneth Clark was a staunch critic of the cultural deprivation theory, warning as early as 1963 of its potential to perpetuate stereotypes of African American inferiority.[13] In his 1965 study of the dy-namics of racial oppression, *Dark Ghetto*, Clark argued that the theory was "seductive." Replacing outmoded theories of biological predeterminism with theories of environmental immutability, cultural deprivation perpetuated negative perceptions of low-income African American children. As deprived children were expected to be incapable of learning, he theorized, no effort was made to teach, thus shifting emphasis from the home lives of African

American children from low-income backgrounds to the educational system that had failed them.[14]

A number of influential critiques of the cultural deprivation approach were published or presented at leading conferences in the late 1960s.[15] By emphasizing the pathological home and family life of individuals from low-income backgrounds, critiques of the cultural deprivation approach argued that this theory was a method of shifting blame and responsibility onto the poor. Sociologist Charles Valentine argued that the War on Poverty was in fact a war on the perceived culture of the poor.[16] Even Riessman, whose work had helped popularize the term, wrote in 1968 that the concept of cultural deprivation was confusing, its meaning and implications were unclear, and it should no longer be considered a useful category of analysis.[17]

By the early 1970s, many scholars had become disillusioned with this theory. In an influential 1970 article, psychologists Stephen and Joan Baratz argued that early childhood enrichment programs based on cultural deprivation theories were in fact a form of institutional racism designed to change and "improve" minorities, focusing on deficiencies rather than on differences.[18] In 1971, psychologist William Ryan described the cultural deprivation theory as an ideology based on "blaming the victim," a term he coined. Arguing that cultural deprivation theory was designed to justify social interventions designed to change not society but society's victim, Ryan ironically described the theory as brilliant.[19] Despite these critiques, many educational theories today continue to draw on the deficit theory of poverty, which finds its roots in the cultural deprivation approach, thus focusing on what is lacking among poor populations.[20]

Matriarchy or Maternal Deprivation?

Much of the theory of cultural deprivation relied on race- and class-specific interpretations of normative mothering and what constituted maternal deprivation. This was certainly not the case in the early descriptions of the "culture of poverty." In Oscar Lewis's 1959 description of "culture of poverty" families, he argued that matrifocality was characteristic particularly of the lower class. Mexican women, although accorded a low social role, held a dominant position within poor families.[21] Among the families he had studied, many fathers were missing, while ties with the mother or "substitute mother figures" were close. Similarly, in *Children of Sanchez*, Lewis again highlighted the trend "toward mother-centered families" and a "great knowledge" of maternal relatives.[22]

Interest in the matrifocal structure of African American families and its relation to the presumed culture of poverty was buoyed by Lewis's descriptions, which circulated widely among American social scientists. Perhaps the culmination of this research was in March 1965, when Daniel Patrick Moynihan, then assistant secretary of labor, submitted to President Johnson a report on African American families, *The Negro Family: A Case for National Action*. Initially secret, this report soon made its way to the media, and it served as the basis for Johnson's June 1965 address at Howard University, in which the president emphasized the "devastating heritage" of slavery for black families.[23] Often referred to simply as the Moynihan Report, this document aroused much controversy and debate, as it portrayed the African American family structure as pathological and as perpetuating the cycle of poverty. The "deterioration of the Negro family" was said to be the "fundamental source of the weakness of the Negro community."[24] Moynihan's report, although guided by a desire to strengthen the African American community, was severely criticized for its judgmental view of black families and its implicit assumptions regarding the superiority of the middle-class Euro-American family.[25] One of the report's main arguments was that the structure of the black family caused a "tangle of pathology" in the African American community. Because black families had historically been headed by women, men did not assume central and traditionally masculine positions in their families. These families, headed by black "matriarchs," could not assist their children in achieving middle-class goals, leading to low scholastic achievement, higher rates of involvement in crime, and psychological difficulties. According to the statistical data Moynihan cited, mainly from U.S. census reports and other governmental reports, black women who functioned as heads of families had more children at an earlier age and higher rates of illegitimacy. Yet they were also better educated than black males, and the majority of these women (56 percent) were employed, earning more money than their male counterparts.[26]

Although Moynihan's presumed family structure accorded black mothers a central role, children in these families were seen as maternally deprived. Having many children prevented mothers from paying adequate attention to each individual child, while the "dependence on the mother's income undermines the position of the father and deprives the children of the kind of attention, particularly in school matters, which is now a standard feature of middle-class upbringing."[27] Thus, by taking on the traditionally masculine role of the breadwinner, African American mothers were in fact causing a unique form of maternal deprivation in their children. Furthermore, black boys fared poorly at school, as their mothers, "disgusted" by male incompetence, encouraged their daughters while neglecting their sons, thus favoring children of the "wrong" gender and further perpetuating this matriarchal pathology.[28] Moynihan's mother-blaming approach relied on psychosocial family theories that highlighted maternal failure as an etiological factor.[29] Thus, even mothers with a significant presence in their children's lives—so significant, in fact, that these women were derogatorily termed "matriarchs"—could be guilty of maternal deprivation when doing so was compatible with the political agenda of the time.

Historian Ruth Feldstein has examined how racialized images of motherhood were enlisted to support liberal ideology. She has compared the attacks on middle-class white "moms," who psychologically damaged their sons by overprotection and overinvolvement, with the images of the black "matriarch" who dominated black men.[30] Contrasting moms and matriarchs, Feldstein argues that liberal social theories highlighting maternal failure followed a strict racial division. Similarly, theories of maternal deprivation took on different forms according to race and class. Middle-class white mothers who chose to work or were overly engaged in their social lives, leaving little time for their children, were seen as guilty of maternal deprivation.[31] Maternal deprivation in low-income African American families took a different form. Black matriarchs who had to seek employment and take on nontraditional gender roles deprived their children of mothers who fulfilled the normative middle-class role, staying at home and assisting with schoolwork. This form of maternal deprivation, to follow Moynihan's argument, lay at the base of the cultural deprivation in African American families.

Though many sociologists and psychologists addressed the prevalence of "matrifocal" families in the African American community, not all of these authors chose to portray such families as maternally deprived.[32] Psychologist Thomas Pettigrew emphasized the dangers of paternal deprivation, while others praised the larger familial and social networks that replaced the nuclear family, thus bringing the children in contact with "uncles, aunties, big mamas, boyfriends, older brothers and sisters."[33] Many sociologists reexamined the same statistical reports as Moynihan but reached contrasting conclusions. Some claimed that matriarchy among the black community was a myth:

Interracial differences in single-parent homes and maternal employment melted away when adjusted according to socioeconomic strata.[34] Yet as the author of one of the major documents that shaped public policy at the time, Moynihan confidently equated matriarchy with maternal deprivation. His interpretation reflected the widespread acceptance of the maternal deprivation theory, which lent further legitimacy to the rising theory of African American disadvantage caused by cultural deprivation.

Oscar Lewis concurred. While Lewis's earlier publications on the culture of poverty had highlighted mothers' central role in family dynamics, by 1966, his view had changed. In the introduction to his 1966 book, *La Vida: A Puerto Rican Family in the Culture of Poverty*, later reprinted in numerous edited volumes, he cited the "high incidence of maternal deprivation, of orality, and of weak ego structure."[35] He had not discovered new data about the family structure; he continued to maintain that these families were led by mothers. Yet Lewis, like Moynihan, embraced the seemingly counterintuitive idea that children who lived in households headed by women were in fact more likely to be maternally deprived because these mothers did not take on the traditional role expected in middle-class families.

Many child development experts shared this view. For example, in an overview of the different compensatory programs available for culturally deprived children, University of Illinois professor of education Celia Stendler-Lavatelli argued that "many mothers are 'bad' mothers because they do not realize that early experiences have an impact upon later development" and do not know how to properly take care of infants. Wedding sensory and maternal deprivation, she suggested that these "culturally deprived" families receive training on how to better stimulate infants.[36] Because mothers were viewed as the mediators of sensory stimulation, cultural deprivation was attributed to a lack of both components.

Some mental health experts used maternal deprivation as a model for understanding cultural deprivation and its long-term effects. The 1962 American Orthopsychiatric Association conference included a panel dedicated to evaluating mental health programs for the "socially deprived," a term often used interchangeably with "culturally deprived." Evaluating the mental health of parents and children from low-income homes, social worker Kermit Wiltse described a prevalent syndrome of "pseudo depression." Characterized by social withdrawal and isolation, inactivity, weight loss, poor appetite, and chronic health problems, this syndrome manifested similarly to clinical depression. The difference was in etiology. Depression, argued Wiltse, "stems from early and severe maternal deprivation" and is "always completely out of proportion to the reality of daily living." In contrast, in these "socially deprived" individuals, the depressive behavior was deemed a "reasonable response" to their "singularly destructive environmental experiences" alongside their "poor ego formation."[37] Hence, the symptoms of depression could be caused by either maternal or social deprivation. In the former case, the damage was psychological and disproportionate to the patient's actual situation; in the latter, the response was appropriate and justified. This formulation also demonstrates how theories of cultural and maternal deprivation were seen as having clinical applicability not only for young children, targeted by compensatory programs, but also for adults. Community mental health workers, Wiltse argued, could treat the psychiatric illnesses caused by deprivation.

Poverty and the Nutritional Metaphor

The cultural deprivation theory of poverty relied on the robust and popularized field of nutritional research. The late nineteenth and early twentieth centuries had seen the isolation of various compounds, later termed vitamins, that were physiologically essential to the human body.[38] These discoveries set the stage for a massive shift in how food was represented in American culture—that is, as having medical and scientific qualities. Nowhere was this change more evident than in the discourse on infant feeding. As historian Rima Apple has argued, mothers, who were traditionally responsible for the diets of their families, were actively involved in the evolution of a scientific discourse on proper infant feeding. The developing science of nutrition had a pivotal role in shaping views of "scientific motherhood"—the belief that mothers should rely on expert scientific and medical advice to raise healthy children—popularized in the early decades of the twentieth century.[39] Mothers sought advice about what foods and feeding schedules were best for infants, and experts provided extremely detailed guidance on the minutiae of infant feeding. Physician Walter Sackett's 1962 *Bringing Up Babies: A Family Doctor's Practical Approach to Child Care*, explained that cereals were allowed on the second day of life, strained vegetables at ten days, strained meat at fourteen days, fruit juice at three weeks, fruit at five weeks, and bacon and eggs for breakfast at nine weeks.[40] Pediatric nutrition was inextricably linked to discussions of normative motherhood, as mothers worked hard to follow inconsistent yet highly demanding expert advice. As Apple has argued, although middle-class white women who did not work had the greatest access to medical pamphlets and child rearing books, the quest for scientific mothering crossed class and racial lines, as low-income and African American women actively sought out such medical information.[41]

By the mid-twentieth century, nutrition was a well-established scientific field. The identification of vitamins and deficiency diseases led to medical breakthroughs, as long-obscure illnesses such as pellagra and pernicious anemia were found to have simple nutritional causes.[42] Nutritionists were confident that many physical ailments and defects could be reduced or even eliminated by correct and balanced feeding. Furthermore, the simplicity of the nutritional deficiency model of disease was compelling; a missing component that could be readily administered made this model widely acceptable and comprehensible to the public. Theories of nutritional deprivation were well established within American culture. In a 1959 Hollywood film, *Operation Petticoat*, a nurse suggested that the hero was "nervous and irritable" because he suffered from a vitamin deficiency.[43] Although most vitamins had been isolated in the early decades of the twentieth century, nutritional research was still being carried out in the 1960s, including work on the interdependence of B_{12} and folic acid. Minerals and trace elements attracted scientific investigation, as did global problems of nutritional deficiency, such as protein deficiency secondary to hunger and famine.[44] Thus, throughout the decade, nutritional research remained a high-profile field of investigation, offering a seemingly simple solution to a host of problems: Provide missing dietary elements.

In the late 1940s, Ancel Keys, a University of Minnesota researcher whose work on starvation had been featured in *Life*, turned his interest from questions of starvation to an analysis of the content of specific diets and their role in illnesses.[45] He designed the Seven Countries Study, a well-known comparative study of diet and illness rates that examined how certain food components correlated with illness. Keys and his collaborators, although later criticized for faulty research methodology, pioneered the study of correlations between high-cholesterol diets and cardiovascular disease. Furthermore, Keys suggested the potential health benefits of what he termed a "Mediterranean diet," arguing that not all diets were equal. In 1959, Keys and his wife published a cookbook accompanied by scientific explanations, *Eat Well and Stay Well*, further shaping public perceptions of nutritional choices as key to healthy living.[46] Key's work on the health risks of fatty foods was featured on the cover of *Time* in 1961, at which point Americans were familiar with the idea that some food elements were essential, some healthy, and some downright dangerous.[47] As nutritional research was described in the popular media, in cookbooks, and in dietary recommendations and as physicians highlighted the importance of proper diet for children and adults alike, it was no wonder that nutrition became a powerful metaphor in American culture.

Within the discourse on cultural deprivation, nutrition served both as a metaphor, reflecting the omnipresence of nutritional discourse in American culture, and as an actual scientific model used to interpret observed clinical data. At times, researchers obliviously used nutrition in both capacities. For example, different early intervention programs, including Head Start, specifically attempted to screen for and eradicate iron deficiency anemia and other deficiency diseases that were seen as characterizing culturally deprived children.[48]

A social worker and researcher at the Social Security Administration, Alvin Schorr, suggested in 1964 that behavior patterns such as lethargy or passivity usually associated with cultural deprivation were in fact physiological outcomes of nutritional deprivation.[49] Citing studies from the 1950s on the effects of malnutrition, including an article by Keys on the effects of starvation, Schorr suggested that symptoms commonly seen as psychological or cultural were in fact the result of malnutrition. Although untrained in medical or nutritional sciences, Schorr, like the nurse in *Operation Petticoat,* thought nutritional deficiencies caused behavioral symptoms. His article, succinctly titled "The Non-Culture of Poverty," rejected the culture of poverty theory. Yet he did not reject the idea that certain behaviors and personality traits characterized the poor; rather, he merely attributed those phenomena to a clear biological cause: nutritional deprivation.

A different use of the nutritional model is evident in University of Tennessee professor of education Ernest Austin's democratic critique of cultural deprivation theory and its translation into public policy. He lamented that money was being spent to reverse the effects of poverty rather than to prevent it. Current approaches to combating cultural deprivation, he argued, were like "movements that come at Christmastime," charity that was inadequately planned and realized. "A child acclimated to a diet of semi-starvation," he argued, could "become deathly ill on a rich feast." This nutritional metaphor was used to criticize the enrichment provided for culturally deprived children, which Austin felt was not always suitable to their needs. Programs designed to alleviate the ravages of poverty and deprivation rather than to change the social structure leading to these conditions were, he claimed, philosophically indefensible. Teachers knew that hungry children could not learn but had only limited ability to provide them with food. Yet even feeding children at school and providing them with education and social interaction would be insufficient, Austin argued. They would emerge from this sheltered school environment unprepared to face the inequalities of American society.[50] Despite being critical of the intervention, Austin accepted the premises of the theory of cultural deprivation, criticizing only the extent of intervention provided. Furthermore, he viewed the model of nutrition as a positive example of how to address cultural deprivation. Like refeeding following starvation, compensatory education had to be informed and measured. Programs countering cultural deprivation, Austin suggested, could be successfully modeled after nutritional enrichment.

Others had a more nuanced view of nutrition as a model for programs designed to counter cultural deprivation. In 1969, while serving as President Nixon's assistant for urban affairs, Moynihan published an edited volume, *On Understanding Poverty*.[51] Looking back at the Johnson administration's War on Poverty, Moynihan was interested in examining what had gone wrong: Why had this promising program failed to attain its goals? Moynihan criticized early government-funded antipoverty programs that failed to examine how the poor were different from others and why and how they could be brought to conform to general society's norms.[52] In the early 1960s, Moynihan argued, policymakers did not take into account the concept of cultural deprivation. The poor had been presumed to be just that: simply poor. No heed was given to the possibility that poverty could effect "structural changes in personality and behavior," just as hunger could lead to malnutrition that could not be resolved by the "resumption of an ample diet."[53] As with prolonged malnutrition, Moynihan reasoned, enrichment could not be accomplished through the simple provision of lacking components. The poor were different; poverty, like malnutrition, led to changes that had to be approached carefully. This analogy framed his view of the necessary structural interventions to remedy long-standing cultural deprivation. His volume, Moynihan promised, would promote a deeper understanding of the ways in which the poor were different and how they could effectively be integrated into majority society.[54]

In contrast, eminent Harvard psychologist Jerome Bruner criticized such attempts to analogize theories of cultural deprivation and compensatory education with theories of nutritional deprivation. He criticized the tendency to view socioeconomic deprivation as a simple deficit, a form of "cultural avitaminosis" to be treated by high doses of compensation. Yet Bruner did not reject the culture of poverty theory, nor did he discredit theories focusing on the dangers of inadequate maternal care. In fact, the main characteristic of the socioeconomic disadvantaged family was the absence or unemployment of the "male wage earner," a viewpoint that echoed theories of the dangers of female-headed families.[55] He criticized a compensatory approach that provided passive enrichment, instead supporting attempts based on community action. Despite Bruner's protests, the nutritional metaphor remained evident in his writing. Elsewhere, he suggested that educational ability could be increased in a variety of ways, depending on the child's preferences and abilities, just as there were many ways of assuring a balanced diet. These different ways reflected local conditions and availability of different diet components; this model could be used, he suggested, to prepare an appropriate program of cultural enrichment.[56] Thus, the model of nutritional supplementation informed his view of early childhood education and methods to improve early achievement.

Other researchers focused on the interplay between nutritional and maternal deprivation, which defined their approach to cultural deprivation. A 1967 article by two physicians and a school administrator in the *American Journal of Clinical Nutrition* examined the health of culturally deprived children. The researchers compared numerous physiological parameters such as height, weight, head circumference, and red blood cell volume among 842 white and African American four-year-olds from low-income homes enrolled in a Baltimore preschool program that served as a forerunner for Project Head Start. Their comparisons showed that African American children were four times as likely to suffer from iron deficiency anemia than their white counterparts. "Disorganized families" had too little meat to feed the children and overrelied on carbohydrates and wheat flour. Furthermore, "misinformed" mothers, they explained, overfed their children milk or used it as a pacifier. Milk further exacerbated the child's anemia, as it was lower in iron than other foods usually given at this age and interfered with iron absorption. Moreover, the irritability and lack of appetite that accompanied anemia could further "disorganize the feeding habits or even the behavior of the mother." The authors therefore argued that "patterns of malnutrition reinforce themselves at both physiologic and social levels."[57] Since anemia was more prevalent among the African American children, these "misinformed" mothers in low-income inner-city homes were in all likelihood African American mothers. This article was based on empirical data and measurements but was shaped by studies of the past decades, which had examined the psychoanalytic significance of feeding behavior. Revealing of the influences on the authors' scholarship was a 1963 article they cited from *Psychosomatic Medicine*. This earlier research had suggested that the "core of the syndrome" of iron deficiency anemia was caused by psychologically unavailable mothers who led their children to turn for comfort to the milk bottle, a phenomenon particularly common in low-income families. The authors of the 1963 article consequently worried about the "development of an oral character crippled more by the nipple of a milk bottle than by a lack of iron."[58]

Analogies between different forms of deprivation and their psychological influences appeared in many articles, as vitamin deficiencies were compared to maternal deprivation and other forms of familial dysfunction.[59] Indeed, some authors referred to a dearth of "intellectual vitamins" suffered by culturally deprived children.[60] Psychologist Lois Murphy described her observations of low-income children participating in different early enrichment programs, mainly in poor urban areas. Although Murphy does not mention the children's race, it can be assumed that at the time, many descriptions of culturally deprived children in the inner cities refer to African American children. These children, she argued, differed from their "well cared-for and stimulated" counterparts. Her entire description was based on metaphors of deprivation:

> Without adequate diets they were too fat or too thin. Without adequate mothering, they were mute, distrustful, inhibited of wildly scattered and screaming. Without an organized home life, they were unable to give sustained attention to work or to play; they were unused to orderly meal-times, a varied diet or the use of spoons, forks etc. . . . Starved for play material, they were hungrily greedy for toys and desperately possessive. They need patient help to understand that the play material would be there day after day for all the children, and they could safely share.[61]

These "culturally deprived" children were in fact depicted as nutritionally and maternally deprived, hungry for food, toys, and personal possessions. The entire interpretation of these children's behavior was based on metaphors of deprivation: starvation, hunger, and lack. Murphy's repeated use of the same sentence structure, with each sentence beginning with what the children lacked as an explanation for their behavior, demonstrates how profoundly theories of deprivation shaped her view of these children and their needs.

Sensory or Cultural Deprivation?

Although various forms of deprivation were subsumed under the description of cultural deprivation, some researchers chose to highlight sensory deprivation. One of the first major discussions of the role of compensatory education in combating cultural deprivation, funded by the Department of Health, Education, and Welfare, took place at a University of Chicago conference in 1964. Organized by distinguished social scientists Benjamin Bloom, Allison Davis, and Robert Hess, the conference's final report was saturated in the sensory deprivation discourse. Although warning against the confusion of organic and cultural deficiencies, the authors claimed that there was little doubt that the two were closely connected.[62] While many African American children were culturally deprived, the report argued, cultural deprivation should not be confused with race, and its recommendations were was deemed relevant for children of all races.[63]

The authors cited the increased incidence of illness, malnutrition, and "gross organ deficiencies" among children of low socioeconomic status. Furthermore, they emphasized the role of "early experiences" in determining readiness for first grade and claimed that the difference between culturally deprived children and their advantaged counterparts lay in the amount and variety of their perceptual experiences. The environment in the deprived child's house provided insufficient stimulation for development both in terms of toys, games, and objects and in terms of the parents, who tended to nod or answer children in monosyllables. In contrast, middle-class children lived in a complex environment with parents who were seen as able to provide more appropriate linguistic stimulation.[64] The lack of sensory stimulation of all forms (auditory, visual, and tactile) in low-income homes was seen to cause a deficit in the children's abilities. Thus compensatory programs were designed to provide what was perceived to be lacking in low-income environments.

Behind the seemingly detached descriptions of the severe sensory deprivation encountered in impoverished homes were often almost outlandish presuppositions of how the "other America" lived. One essay described a little boy who was said to have difficulties distinguishing between a picture of a pig and a picture of a little girl, presumably because of a lack of exposure to visual stimulation.[65] Another researcher, echoing sensory deprivation terminology, claimed that the deficiencies in speech among culturally deprived children resulted from the "more restricted nature of the environment" in which they were raised. She explained that "reliance upon language as a means of effective communication as well as cognitive exploration is particularly prevalent in the small, nuclear middle-class home," a statement that raises questions regarding how she imagined communication in non-middle-class homes might take place.[66] Indeed, as Edward Zigler and Karen Anderson aptly wrote in their 1979 critique of the cultural deprivation theory, descriptions of communication in impoverished families left the impression that poor people did not speak at all but rather gesticulated, grunted, or shouted.[67] This stereotype was deeply ingrained. In fact, researchers worried about what would happen following early intervention: Would low-income parents even be able to deal with their children's increased verbal communication? Psychologist Joseph McVicker Hunt wrote to Lois Murphy that parents of children who had attended early enrichment programs developed ambivalent feelings: They were "proud of the capacity of their children to talk, but they are troubled by the amount of talk that they have to listen to."[68]

Hunt was one of the main scientific figures involved in promoting the theory of cultural deprivation. A psychology professor at the University of Illinois and past president of the American Psychology Association, Hunt was particularly interested in child development and early education.[69] His 1961 book, *Intelligence and Experience,* was widely seen as heralding a new and environmentally focused theoretical approach to the development of intelligence. In his often-cited article published three years later, "The Psychological Basis for Using Preschool Enrichment as an Antidote for Cultural Deprivation," Hunt gave an important theoretical impetus to child psychologists and development experts who developed early enrichment programs, establishing himself as an expert in the field despite his lack of practical experience. After extensively citing sensory deprivation experiments on animals and humans, Hunt claimed that the difference between culturally deprived children and their privileged counterparts was "analogous to the difference between cage-reared and pet-reared rats and dogs." Although he admitted that this notion of cultural deprivation was "gross and undifferentiated," Hunt did not hesitate to endorse the practical implications of his theory in the form of early preschool intervention.[70] This parallel between animals and children was made abundantly clear at the close of the article, where Hunt stated that he "viewed the effects of cultural deprivation as analogous to the experimentally found effects of experiential deprivation in infancy."[71]

Significantly, while Hunt was aware of the limitations of his theorization on cultural deprivation and its possible antidote (preschool enrichment), his prestige and publications led others to believe that the volume of evidence available was far larger than it in fact was. Urie Bronfenbrenner, a psychologist and child development expert at Cornell University, wrote Hunt to request references to Hunt's work on cultural deprivation. Familiar with Hunt's research, Bronfenbrenner had been surprised by a colleague serving as a consultant on public welfare who had cited Hunt's work as demonstrating that it was possible to raise the learning level of children from culturally deprived environments. Admitting embarrassment at his unfamiliarity with this research, Bronfenbrenner requested that Hunt send reprints.[72] Hunt responded that while the term "demonstration usually implies empirical work," he had completed no such research, although he had written a number of theoretical articles on the topic. These articles, which Hunt described as "surveying the evidence" on the topic, were based on sensory deprivation research and early observations on maternal deprivation.[73] Once again, empirical evidence regarding the nature of cultural deprivation was assumed to be available and was cited by and exchanged among politicians and experts. In fact, however, no such data existed; these theoretical pronouncements rested only on new interpretations of old data on sensory and maternal deprivation.

Although Hunt's work was solely theoretical, he was still viewed as a source of expert practical knowledge. Preschool educators wrote to ask him a broad variety of questions, citing his expertise in combating cultural deprivation. One educator wondered whether to buy a tricycle or a merry-go-round, while mothers were interested in possible enrichment activities for their children.[74] In the face of this widespread enthusiasm and endorsement of his ideas, Hunt expressed concern about the rapid acceptance of preschool enrichment as a means to combat cultural deprivation, warning against the development of programs based on insufficient data.[75] Attempting to maintain his position of scientific authority, Hunt urged caution and highlighted the need for further research before establishing large-scale enrichment programs. Yet instead of leading to a questioning of the available evidence on cultural deprivation, this guarded position only strengthened the assumption that such evidence was abundantly available and further established Hunt as an authority in cultural deprivation research.

Linguistic Deprivation, Bernstein, and Labov

Sociolinguistic theories were closely tied to research on cultural deprivation, as researchers evaluated the mother-child interaction and how it shaped models of language acquisition. American researchers commonly portrayed low-income and African American mothers as speaking in monosyllables, impeding their children's attempts to verbally express themselves and discouraging their natural curiosity. These researchers relied on the work of British sociologist and linguist Basil Bernstein, although he did not share their judgmental assumptions.

In the early stages of his graduate work in linguistics at University College London, Bernstein developed what was to become an enormously influential theory in the emerging field of sociolinguistics, which examines how society and its norms govern linguistic interaction. In 1962, he published two seminal articles that outlined his theory of codes and distinguished between what he defined as restricted and elaborated code.[76] He defined codes according to the "probability of predicting for any one speaker which structural elements will be used to organise meaning." In the case of an elaborated code, the speaker could select elements from an extensive range of alternatives, so the ability to predict was low. In the restricted code, the alternatives were limited, so the ability to predict was increased. The restricted code was used in particular social settings, such as in religious or social ceremonies, or limited interactions, from conversations on the weather to the mundane dialogue of a married couple negotiating whose turn it was to put the kettle on and walk the dog.[77] The elaborated code was complete and universal; it did not require background knowledge of context or details. It highlighted individual style and facilitated the verbal transmission and elaboration of the individual's unique experience. Although a restricted code would be appropriate in numerous life situations, Bernstein generalized that working-class families spoke mainly in restricted code, whereas middle-class families often spoke in elaborated code. Bernstein stressed that both codes were useful, depending on context.

Bernstein's early publications had referred to the differences between the codes middle- and lower-class parents used when speaking to their children. These class differences in parent-child interaction soon became the central focus of his research, although they were not necessarily his primary interest. Pressure exerted by the University of London Institute of Education, his funding institution, led Bernstein specifically to examine how young infants and toddlers interacted with their parents. Although he had originally planned to examine children's language from the nursery through age fifteen, he soon narrowed his research to parent-child interactions at the early end of that range.[78]

As Bernstein's work gained international attention, prominent researchers used his code theory as the theoretical basis for examining their own research hypotheses. Most noteworthy is the interaction between Bernstein and University of Chicago professor of psychology Robert Hess. While attending a 1963 conference at the University of Chicago, Bernstein met Hess, who was conducting research on maternal teaching styles and communication. Hess had an active interest in theories of deprivation and compensation and was one of the organizers of the 1964 University of Chicago conference on compensatory education. The two men admired each other's work.[79]

In 1965, Hess and his colleague, Virginia Shipman, used Bernstein's code theory to devise an experiment examining the language used by mothers in speaking to their children, focusing on 163 African American women of different socioeconomic backgrounds and their four-year-old children. Their experiment was formulated to answer the question "What is cultural deprivation, and how does it act to shape and depress the resources of the human mind?"[80] This question expressed their acceptance of the theory of cultural deprivation and its role in impeding scholastic achievement. Their study analyzed mother-child interactions among four groups of mothers divided according to education and socioeconomic status. The mothers were asked to assist their children in a block-sorting task and in drawing a shape on an Etch-a-Sketch toy. The researchers examined the interaction between mother and child, focusing on the words and sentence structures mothers used to encourage and assist their children. The researchers argued that mothers from middle-class backgrounds could guide their children more effectively than low-income mothers, who had difficulties explaining the tasks to their children. Thus, the main characteristic of cultural deprivation the researchers found was "a lack of cognitive meaning in the mother-child communication system." Utilizing theories of linguistic deprivation, they concluded that the "meaning of deprivation is a deprivation of meaning" within the mother-child interaction, which ultimately framed and impeded the child's cognitive growth and development.[81] When the mother-child interaction is deprived of meaning, cultural deprivation ensues.

Bernstein's work was quickly adapted in the experiments and interventions designed by researchers interested in different forms of deprivation. Psychologist Carl Bereiter and his University of Illinois colleagues similarly relied on their erroneous view of Bernstein's theory as they devised an intervention designed to teach African American children to speak Standard English. A highly contested term, Standard English refers to the variety of English spoken mainly by educated individuals (as opposed to regional

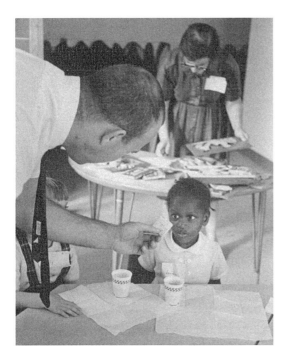

Siegfried Engelmann and a four-year-old student at the University of Illinois intervention program headed by Carl Bereiter. Photo by Leonard McCombe. Courtesy of Time & Life Pictures/Getty Images.

dialects) and is the language taught to non-English-speakers.[82] Bereiter's "academically oriented" preschool program, unlike other interventions that emphasized only educational play activities, specifically targeted language acquisition. Bereiter claimed that his study's intervention followed Bernstein's view of nonstandard English as "not merely an underdeveloped version of standard English" but a "non-logical mode of expressive behavior," a view Bernstein had never expressed and later publicly rejected.[83] Bereiter and his colleagues held such negative views of the children's linguistic capacities that they argued that it was best to approach these children as though they had "no language at all."[84] Clearly biased against the speech of African American children, the researchers argued that it was deficient in logic, even when it seemed clear that it was not. For example, they considered "Me got juice" to be a "series of badly connected words"; "in the tree" was considered an incorrect response to the question "Where is the squirrel?" The correct answer was "The squirrel is in the tree," and children were drilled to answer in complete sentences. Like Hess before him, Bereiter and his colleagues used Bernstein's linguistic theories as the basis for interventions targeting perceived deprivations; these children were seen to be so deprived that Bereiter compared them to deaf children.[85]

In 1966, Bernstein participated in a symposium on "Perspectives on Learning" at the Bank Street College of Education in New York; his expenses were underwritten by the Ford Foundation. In his presentation on the role of speech in the development and transmission of culture, Bernstein argued that there was no easy way to prevent the "indignity of social class from marking the experience of a child"; there were no tips or interventions "to which we can expose a child and jack up his IQ by thirteen points."[86] This was a tongue-in-cheek critique of early intervention programs that promised far more than they could possibly deliver, including mitigating the detrimental effects of poverty and prejudice. Thus, Bernstein began his presentation by expressing his reservations about the use of his work as the theoretical basis for early intervention programs. He repeatedly highlighted the value of the restricted code and demonstrated different situations—particularly mundane exchanges—in which it would be the only appropriate form of speech. "God help the man that can't use a restricted code," Bernstein quipped; "his wife must find it very painful."[87]

Reflecting debates about the language of low-income and African American children, Bernstein emphatically argued that "it is a whole lot of nonsense to speak of a nonverbal child," although the child might seem to be inarticulate in a certain social context. He repeatedly emphasized that the codes were not a value judgment in themselves.[88]

In describing his research findings, he demonstrated how mothers from different class backgrounds use different codes to exert control over their children. Using a restricted code, for example, would be saying, "Do it because I say so"; an elaborate code would be, "I know you don't like to kiss Grandpa, but he's very fond of you and it makes him happy."[89] Hence, the restricted code was positional and based on the power relations between the mother and the child, whereas the elaborated code was personal. Middle-class mothers more often used elaborate code with their children, which led, Bernstein argued, to a more complicated relationship between child and parents. Yet a more complicated relationship was not an unmitigated good, Bernstein warned: "It is not unusual for people who use an elaborated code to be constantly preoccupied with who they are, with problems of identity."[90]

For Bernstein, the elaborated code was not a better form of communication than the restricted code. Rather, his linguistic research examined the social significance of the different codes and their uses. He clarified his approach during the ensuing discussion, when he was asked whether an elaborated code was not more psychologically advanced than the restricted code.

Bernstein answered with questions of his own: Was making love a regressed behavior? Was going out for drinks and letting "our hair down" regressed behavior? Bernstein argued that each behavior—and similarly, each code—was appropriate in certain contexts.[91]

When asked by Mario Fantini, program officer for the Ford Foundation Fund for the Advancement of Education, about how Bernstein's model could be used to approach what Fantini termed the "problem of deprivation," Bernstein answered in no uncertain terms: "This notion of treating children as exhibiting various kinds of deficits turns the social scientist into a plumber whose task is to plug, or rather fill, the deficits," he argued. When viewing the child "as a cognitive or perceptual deficit," the educator loses sight of the "vital nature of the communal experience of the child and the many cultural and psychological processes at work in him."[92] His work, Bernstein explained, was in fact a critique of the deficit theory, calling for a more comprehensive understanding of the different processes involved in particular social situations. Bernstein thus openly criticized the approach taken by the senior educator and administrator of the foundation that had paid for his participation in the conference.

Yeshiva University professor of education Vera John warned of Americans' "vulgarization" of Bernstein's theories through simplistic attempts to correlate between social class and code. Furthermore, John argued, the disadvantaged groups examined by American researchers were heterogenic. The lower working class in England, she argued, did not display the same characteristics as third-generation Polish families or "Mississippi delta Negro families" in the United States and could not be expected to demonstrate the same linguistic features. John argued that during a period of "social movement and cultural growth," the civil rights movement, African Americans in Mississippi showed linguistic "force and beauty" despite their limited "competence in articulation."[93]

Bernstein agreed with John that groups limited to a restricted code could still "change their social position, their civil rights, through social action." Still, he argued, society purposely used the class system to create the situation in which disenfranchised groups most often use restricted code and thus were cut off "from the power of intellectual criticism." Accordingly, the use of codes, he argued, was a method of social control.[94] In response to John's description of the American vulgarization of his theories, Bernstein vigorously defended Hess's research, emphasizing that references to the "vulgar Bernstein model" should not include Hess's work.[95] Both Bernstein and

John chose not to mention any other specific research program as indicative of a "vulgarized" Bernstein approach. However, Bereiter's work, published the same year in which the symposium was held, was the most prominent other research program of the time being carried out ostensibly on the basis of Bernstein's theory. Although Bernstein expressed less concern than John about this oversimplification of his theory, he soon changed his tune, particularly in light of criticism voiced by a rising young linguist, William Labov.

After completing his dissertation at Columbia University in 1964 on the different language forms used by New Yorkers, Labov began a project, funded by the U.S. Office of Education, examining the language of African American schoolchildren in Harlem. He was interested in assessing whether their dialect explained their difficulties in reading. Motivated by a strong sense of social justice, Labov later described his efforts as designed to counter institutionalized racism and prejudice against African Americans and their speech patterns.[96] He interviewed members of gangs in Harlem, most famously the Cobras and the Jets, to assess the influence of what he termed "peer group status" on reading skills.[97]

At the time, little work had been carried out on what is known today as African American Vernacular English (AAVE), and linguists debated whether it was a creole, with English vocabulary superimposed on African grammar, or a regional dialect. In contrast, many white educators and psychologists such as Bereiter and his colleagues viewed AAVE as simply a form of faulty English. Its speakers were even deemed "nonverbal" and their language described as illogical. The pattern of double negatives ("He don't know nothing") was considered evidence of faulty logic by Anglocentric speakers of Standard English, who might not have been aware that the double negative was the correct form in numerous languages.[98]

At a 1969 linguistic conference in Washington, D.C., Labov presented what became a seminal essay, "The Logic of Nonstandard English."[99] His findings indicated that AAVE had distinct grammatical structure and rules and was not simply flawed English. Furthermore, Labov argued that the language of the African American youth he had interviewed was rich and reflected clear logical thinking. Labov criticized Bernstein on the grounds that his views were "filtered through a strong bias against all forms of working-class behavior, so that middle-class language is seen as superior in every respect." Yet Labov did not engage directly with Bernstein's work. Rather, his criticism was directed toward Bereiter and his colleagues' descriptions of the language of young African American children. He cited Bereiter's claim that the language of "cultural deprived children" was "not merely an underdeveloped version of Standard English" but was a basically "non-logical mode of expressive behavior." Although most linguists and psycholinguists would simply view this contention as "utter nonsense," Labov argued, he focused on how Bereiter's team had reached these conclusions. Labov claimed that their work was hinged on observations carried out in an asymmetrical testing situation in which the child answered in defensive, monosyllabic language, knowing that "anything he says can literally be held against him."[100] When interactions were conducted by experienced interviewers who were familiar with the community and with the children they were interviewing, the results differed significantly: The children spoke at length, displaying rich language.[101]

Thus for Labov, the "view of the Negro speech community" that arose from his research contrasted starkly with that of Bereiter and his like-minded colleagues. Where they had seen language deficits among low-income, African American children, Labov described a "child bathed in verbal stimulation from morning to night." Furthermore, Labov questioned the assumption of the superiority of the "elaborated code," suggesting that it was often "turgid, redundant and empty" and was simply a style rather than a code or system of thought.[102]

Labov's paper is considered groundbreaking in the field of sociolinguists and has been reprinted numerous times since it was first presented in 1969, including a version that reached a wide readership in the *Atlantic Monthly* in 1972.[103] It provided a comprehensive analysis of the workings of AAVE as a dialect of American English, severely criticizing theories that held African American children to be deficient in their ability to express themselves logically. Labov's paper also had an influential role in shaping how Bernstein's theories would eventually come be viewed, pitting Bernstein and Labov in opposition to each other as representative of two opposing camps: deficit versus difference. Although Labov later admitted that he had not read Bernstein's work but had based his critique on the interpretation of Bernstein as reflected by the works of Bereiter and Engelmann and others, his negative portrayal of Bernstein's work had a lasting impression.[104]

Ironically, much of Labov's work can be seen as concurring with and even strengthening Bernstein's arguments. Labov extensively cited verbatim dialogues, which he later broke up into logical arguments, in effect translating the material from restricted to elaborated code. He further elaborated the cultural context to elucidate the vocabulary used. He explained, for example, that in the context of black nationalism, the term "po'k chop God" was a derogatory reference to the traditional God of Southern Baptists, whose followers had not yet embraced an empowering Muslim ideology.[105] These acts of translation and elaboration can be seen as confirming Bernstein's theory of a restricted code in action.[106]

Labov grouped Bernstein, who had been one of the earliest critics of cultural deprivation, with the deficit theorists, a designation from which he later worked hard to distance himself. While in 1966, Bernstein had only feebly concurred with Vera John's disapproval of the "vulgarization" of his work, in his 1971 book, *Class, Code, and Control*, he dedicated an entire chapter to the critique of the concept of compensatory education. He argued that these compensatory programs directed attention away from the deficiencies of the school and instead focused on deficiencies in the community, family, and child.[107] In the second revised edition of the book, published in 1974, Bernstein directly engaged with Labov's criticism in "The Logic of Nonstandard English," answering each of Labov's specific criticisms with citations from his own publications and thus demonstrating how closely aligned the two men's approaches were. Bernstein then cited his response to Mario Fantini's question on cultural deprivation at the 1966 Bank Street conference, which he described as one of the "first public critiques of the deficit thesis."[108]

By the late 1960s and early 1970s, Bernstein was prepared to fight back against Labov's criticism. Yet Bernstein's reputation, at least among nonlinguists not directly familiar with his work, was tainted. A friend and former student described in Bernstein's obituary how he had been called a "fascist" by an anthropologist who had never read his work.[109]

Although Bernstein rejected the deprivation hypothesis, cultural deprivation theorists in the United States, among them Robert Hess, relied on Bernstein's work to provide seemingly scientific evidence for their theories. Using Bernstein's theory of code, American researchers merged two forms of deprivation, maternal and sensory, to create the linguistic deprivation theory, though it was far from Bernstein's original theory of codes. This theory held that low-income and African American mothers had limited verbal capacities that impeded their children's intellectual and linguistic development. Furthermore, as these mothers spoke in monosyllables and often quieted their children rather than encouraging them to speak, this behavior created a form of sensory deprivation. The result was cultural deprivation, which, as Hess had argued, meant the "deprivation of meaning" in the mother-child relationship.[110] Thus, linguistic deprivation, a component of cultural deprivation, was also based on race- and class-specific interpretations of maternal and sensory deprivation.

Criticism within the Deprivation Framework

During the 1960s, although the theory of cultural deprivation and its reliance on sensory deprivation studies were widely accepted, a number of psychologists and sociologists questioned whether young children growing up in impoverished households truly suffered from deprivation and if they did, until what age. Yet even within this debate, no distinction was made between cultural and sensory deprivation. Until the early 1970s, Hunt, a vocal supporter of the cultural deprivation theory, often expressed his opinion that low-income home environments were not depriving for young infants but were depriving only for toddlers, who needed more stimulation from their environment when they began to walk. He argued that culturally deprived children differed greatly from those reared in orphanages, rejecting attempts to tie René Spitz's early description of the dangers of infant institutionalization and the later descriptions of cultural deprivation. In fact, Hunt argued that for young infants, life in impoverished settings could offer an "enriched environment," full of stimulation in the form of the sights and smells of a crowded apartment.[111] Yet in the second year of life, the same crowding that had originally afforded adequate stimulation now provided a paucity of playthings and models for imitation. Relying on physiological studies, Hunt compared the effects of the restricted environment during different periods of infancy to the case of tadpoles and young chicks. In the early period, they did not seem to suffer from a restricted environment, but if these conditions continued, their swimming abilities or pecking responses were irreversibly hampered.[112]

Hunt's criticism resembled that voiced by scholars who completely rejected the cultural deprivation approach. In a book designed to expose the "myth" of the deprived child, Columbia University professor of education and psychology Herbert Ginsburg argued that no evidence showed that "the slum is not a stimulating environment in its own way" since it contained sounds, shapes, and obstacles to surmount, relying on the wealth of sensory stimulation to argue against the existence of cultural deprivation.[113] Kenneth Clark, a longtime critic of the cultural deprivation theory, argued for what he termed a more "parsimonious" theory. African American children from low-income homes did not succeed at school because they were expected to fail and insufficient effort was made to teach them. Cultural deprivation had been "made synonymous with stimulus deprivation," Clark argued, and urban, working-class African American children were seen as having "absolutely no sensory stimulation."[114] He, too, rejected this perception of impoverished homes as lacking in sensory stimulation, but he did not question the generally accepted correlation between the availability of sensory stimulation and cultural deprivation. Even Clark and the other vocal critics of the cultural deprivation approach did not challenge the parallels among maternal, sensory, and cultural deprivation. In fact, their attempts to disprove the theory of cultural deprivation often relied on demonstrations that there was no evidence of sensory or maternal deprivation.

Deprivation and the Nature-Nurture Debate

The years following the U.S. Supreme Court's 1954 ruling against school segregation, *Brown v. Board of Education,* saw a resurgence of the old debate regarding whether intelligence was determined by environment or heredity. While theories of intelligence highlighting hereditary differences between the races had been accepted in American scientific culture in the early decades of the twentieth century, the wake of World War II saw a significant decline in the acceptability of such theories. Faced with the prospect of desegregated southern schools, white southern scientists—anatomists, psychologists, and others—as well as politicians took up the argument that African Americans were intellectually inferior.[115] Proponents of this view attempted to discredit the works of antiracist scientists by appealing to white southern "common sense" and eliciting fears of a liberal and often Jewish conspiracy. White southerners' personal knowledge of racial differences was accorded a privileged role in this debate.[116]

The crux of this debate centered on scholastic tests designed to measure academic aptitude and intelligence, on which African American children scored lower than European American children.[117] This discrepancy in test scores, known as the racial achievement gap, had been described from the early decades of the twentieth century.[118] While segregationist scientists such as psychologist Audrey Shuey attributed this gap to the innate intellectual inferiority of African American children, antiracist scientists, liberal politicians, and African American researchers were developing an entirely different set of hypotheses and interpretations. The low quality of the schools attended by black children, substandard teachers, home environment and family situation, and in particular poverty and its ramifications were all seen as important causes of this test score gap.[119] Segregationist scientists dismissed these theories, reaffirming their views of white superiority.[120] Yet by 1964, with the passage of the Civil Rights Act, their works fell into disrepute, and segregationist views became far less common and influential than they had been in the previous decade.[121] Furthermore, by the mid-1960s, observers began to question the relevance of standardized tests to minority communities, and many minority leaders called for a complete rejection of these forms of testing. In 1968, the newly established Association of Black Psychologists called for a moratorium on the testing of black children until an appropriately culturally sensitive test was developed. This move further intensified public debates regarding intelligence testing.[122] Thus, researchers began to question the existence of the racial gap as well as whether it indeed reflected minority children's abilities.

In the early 1960s, the scientific community shifted its emphasis to the environmental determinants of intellectual performance. Two books in particular—*Intelligence and Experience* (1961) by Joseph McVicker Hunt and *Stability and Change in Human Characteristics* (1964) by educational psychologist Benjamin Bloom—have been credited as providing the scientific and intellectual basis for the environmental approach.[123] Hunt highlighted the importance of early experiences in the shaping of intelligence and psychological development; Bloom claimed that intelligence could be modified by experience in the first five years of life, after which it became relatively resistant to environmental influence. Both books accorded a central role to the findings of sensory deprivation experiments in shaping their theories of intelligence, as well as the findings of René Spitz and other early studies on institutionalized children, particularly in orphanages.[124] While both Bloom and Hunt argued that experience shaped intelligence, they based their work on studies that had examined how different forms of deprivation suppressed intellectual ability. Thus, deprivation experiments provided much of the scientific evidence cited in both books.

Based on Bloom's and Hunt's claims that intelligence was shaped by experience, educational researchers argued that a dearth of experiences would necessarily lead to depressed intellectual development. Providing additional experiences in the form of early childhood enrichment, it stood to reason, would increase intellectual ability. Bloom's and Hunt's books were seen as proof of the detrimental intellectual effects of deprivation and were cited extensively throughout the 1960s, including in descriptions of the scientific rationale for programs such as Project Head Start.[125] Studies examining sensory and maternal deprivation consequently were co-opted into the accepted scientific rationale for an environmentalist approach to the development of intelligence and served as the theoretical basis for early intervention programs.

Deprivation-based approaches were commonly invoked to explain the racial gap in scholastic tests. In 1964, Thomas Pettigrew, a white antiracist psychologist who became an expert on African American society, published "Negro American Intelligence: A New Look at an Old Controversy." This influential essay was later reprinted in his monograph, *A Profile of the Negro American*, seen at the time as an authoritative study of African American psychology.[126] Pettigrew began his essay by analyzing the surge in what he termed "scientific racism" following the *Brown* decision. He criticized researchers who did not pay adequate attention to the role of socioeconomic status, which he argued was never completely matched in studies comparing between white and African American children. Accordingly, until segregation and discrimination were completely abolished, no "definitive research on racial differences in intelligence" could be performed. While in previous decades, the debate could be conceptualized as simply a question of nature versus nurture, current studies examine the interplay between environment and heredity.[127] He demonstrated this argument through a description of an experiment carried out by sensory deprivation researcher John Zubek on two strains of rats, bright and dull. These two groups were distinguished on the basis of experiments from the early 1940s in which rats were bred according to their ability to navigate mazes.[128] Zubek kept the rats in three different environments: a deprived environment, an enriched environment, and one said to provide "normal" stimulation. The rats performed equally well in the deprived and in the enriched environments; only in the "normal" environment did their learning ability differ. This, Pettigrew argued, was evidence of the interplay between environment and genetics: The environment could mask and obliterate hereditary differences. Pettigrew also cited Hunt's work to argue that intelligence was not a genetically predetermined trait but rather a "dynamic, on-going set of processes that within wide hereditary limits is subject to innumerable experiential factors."[129] Thus, while heredity set limits on intellectual development, the realization of this potential was mediated through the environment.

Pettigrew cited a list of deprivation-based experiments as evidence for the validity of an environmentalist approach to the development of intelligence. These experiments included early education programs with children seen to suffer from an intellectual disability, the gain in IQ of orphans in institutions following their adoption into loving homes, and studies pointing to an inverse relationship between family size and intelligence. These studies, he argued, demonstrated that children with many siblings did not fare as well as children raised in smaller families because they received less individual stimulation from their parents. Vitamin and iron deficiencies were cited as additional causes of underdeveloped intelligence, as Pettigrew referred to studies of the effects of nutritional enrichment.[130] Pettigrew also drew on the work of psychologist Martin Deutsch, who had described how "lower-class youngsters in a ghetto school" (African American students in Harlem neighborhoods) had never ventured more than twenty-five blocks from their homes. For them, Pettigrew argued, echoing theories of cultural deprivation, the school was a "foreign outpost in an encapsulated community." Finally, Pettigrew cited the "extreme effects" of an "impoverished environment" as demonstrated by experiments in sensory deprivation.[131] In rejecting the hereditarian theory of white intellectual superiority, Pettigrew relied heavily on theories of deprivation. He viewed emotional deprivation by parents, sensory deprivation, cultural deprivation, and nutritional deficits as putative causes of interracial differences in intelligence. Rejecting claims of hereditary interracial differences in innate intelligence, Pettigrew relied on different theories of deprivation to interpret the black-white score gap in scholastic testing. Pettigrew's influential essay, often cited as a comprehensive rebuttal of segregationist scientists' claims, is a clear example of how psychologists adopted and utilized deprivation theories to advance antiracist views of interracial differences.

While antiracist scholars such as Pettigrew relied on deprivation theories, deprivation experts incorporated their support of the civil rights movement into their work, a process that at times required considerable effort in order to reconcile their commitment to deprivation theory and their political leanings. Psychologist and maternal deprivation expert Mary Ainsworth described her mixed feelings at the compensatory education movement. For years she had accepted John Bowlby's view that institutional care, including day care programs, risked causing maternal deprivation in infants. Yet in a letter to Bowlby, she described her strong support of the civil rights movement, arguing that "the negro is inferior only through deprivation—cultural and maternal." The only way to address this deprivation quickly was "to do something massive about children."[132] Although she worried about possible maternal deprivation that could be caused by early enrichment programs that provided care for young infants away from their mothers, her commitment to civil rights led her to accept the necessity of such programs.

Although deprivation theories were embraced primarily by researchers who believed that intelligence was determined by the environment, they were also adopted by proponents of a hereditarian approach. Some researchers postulated a genetic and race-based predisposition or vulnerability to certain forms of deprivation. In a 1967 *Science* article examining experiential deprivation in dogs, physiologist James Fuller claimed that it was widely accepted that early sensory and motor deprivation was responsible for "a considerable portion of mental retardation and social inadequacy" in humans.[133] The article compared the effects of varying degrees of deprivation on two different breeds of dogs, with parameters designed to reflect the dogs' learning ability and social behavior. The results of the experimental deprivation were inconsistent: Some dogs raised in isolation performed well, while others performed poorly. Fuller concluded that deprivation did not necessarily prevent the development of normal intelligence but was detrimental to the performance of vulnerable individuals. Thus, he suggested that vulnerability to deprivation had a genetically determined component; it did not affect everyone equally. Fuller also explored the possible social and political implications of this experiment for humans, describing the "environmental impoverishment" of urban, low-income home life as on par with experimental sensory deprivation. While most subjects emerged unscathed, the genetically vulnerable individual would suffer from impeded intellectual development.[134] In this manner, Fuller incorporated the theory of deprivation to further a hereditarian theory of vulnerability: Some "breeds" were more vulnerable than others.

A similar view can be found in a 1969 article in the *American Mercury*, a journal identified with racist and anti-Semitic opinions and supported by the Pioneer Fund, a foundation dedicated to encouraging research on the genetics and heredity of intelligence.[135] This article asked, "Why aren't Indians 'disadvantaged?'" Robert Kuttner, a biologist and self-described proponent of "scientific racism," highlighted the socioeconomic disadvantages of Native Americans as well as their racial oppression. Yet despite such adverse living conditions, Kuttner argued, the scholastic achievement of Native American children was consistently higher than that of their African American counterparts. This was evidence, he claimed, for the importance of genetic explanations for the racial achievement gap, as environmental factors could no longer be viewed as "totipotent." While using the word "disadvantage" rather than "deprivation," Kuttner referred to the "environmental handicaps" he claimed were commonly invoked to explain the achievement gap.[136] By highlighting the environmental disadvantage of Native Americans, Kuttner relied on the same premises accepted by environmentalists: a belief that a deprived environment led to lower scholastic achievement. Yet Kuttner did so to further his hereditarian position, using theories of environmental deprivation to argue for the innate intellectual inferiority of African Americans. Although certainly not an influential publication, this article demonstrates how even clearly racist scientists incorporated deprivation theory in their arguments.

The Jensen Debate

The year 1969 signified a turning point in the debate over the nature of racial differences. In January 1969, Richard Nixon assumed office, a Republican president chosen after Americans had grown increasingly disillusioned with Johnson's presidency and in particular the Vietnam War, for which no satisfactory end seemed to be in sight. Furthermore, the urban race riots of the decade had led many liberal white Americans to rethink their continued support of the civil rights movement, which had taken on militarist and separationist characteristics far from the late Martin Luther King Jr.'s palatable and pacifist agenda.[137] Some liberals had become disenchanted by both the civil rights movement and the War on Poverty, seeing these programs as efforts to excessively empower the black community. Many experienced the race riots as a personal affront. Nixon thus rode into office on a wave of white backlash.[138]

The year 1969 also saw the publication of the Westinghouse Learning Cooperation Report, an evaluation of Project Head Start commissioned by the U.S. Office of Economic Opportunity that ultimately found few long-term differences between children who had participated in the program and those who had not.[139] Such findings raised a vigorous debate regarding the effectiveness of early enrichment programs. In the same year, University of California at Berkeley professor of psychology Arthur Jensen published a highly controversial and widely cited article in the *Harvard Educational Review*, "How Much Can We Boost IQ and Scholastic Achievement?," in which he argued for a hereditary component of intelligence.[140] Jensen's article played an important role in revitalizing a debate that effectively had been set aside since the mid-1960s. The article provided a theoretical underpinning for the arguments of segregationist scientists and was celebrated by champions of white supremacy. Many psychologists who espoused theories of racial difference welcomed Jensen's argument that political concerns had hitherto prevented a thorough, scientific evaluation of race, thus presenting their hereditarian approach to science as a victim of liberal politics.

Presenting his work as "real" science, Jensen depicted himself as a maverick, unimpeded by the constraints of political correctness. Since the publication of the article, Jensen has consistently denied his support for segregation and has rejected the enlistment of his research to support this cause.[141] Despite his protests, as historian John P. Jackson has argued, Jensen's claim that his work was rejected not because of its scientific value but because of its unpopular political implications unwittingly echoed the conspiracy theories of segregation scientists during the 1950s.[142]

In 1968, Jensen had published a shorter article mapping out the same basic arguments as part of an edited volume on Head Start and early intervention. In this lesser-known article, he examined the debate over the determinants of intelligence and suggested analogizing the role of "environmental stimulation" with the effects of nutritional variance: If the minimal physiological requirements were lacking, growth would be impeded. Conversely, no amount of vitamins and minerals could increase a well-nourished individual's stature. For Jensen, this analogy seemed so self-evident that he did not cite a single study examining the relation between nutrition and human development; he assumed that his readers shared his understanding of the interaction between environment and genetics in the case of nutrition. Furthermore, Jensen argued that extreme sensory deprivation might lower a child's IQ, but it could be boosted by moving the child to an adequate environment. However, he claimed, beyond a certain threshold, differences in stimulation had negligible effects on IQ.[143] In this case, the analogy between nutritional and sensory deprivation was used to discredit and criticize the cultural deprivation approach, setting the ground for his 1969 rejection of compensatory education and his support for the hereditary basis of intelligence.

In his often-cited 1969 article, Jensen claimed that compensatory education had been tried and "apparently it had failed," suggesting a reevaluation of the premises of early enrichment programs. He based this argument on the different evaluations of Head Start and in particular on the Westinghouse Report, which had failed to find a significant increase in intellectual ability following compensatory enrichment. Jensen's article, denounced by many as racist, argued that racial differences in scholastic achievement as measured by performance on standardized tests resulted at least partially from genetic factors. This view was singularly unpopular at the end of the 1960s. Interpretation of the racial gap in test performance formed part of a heated debate over strategies for improving educational opportunities for minority children. Theories that presented the home environments of African American children as detrimental to intellectual development proposed intervention programs providing early childhood enrichment. Liberal educators who faulted the crowded classrooms and impoverished facilities of segregated schools presented desegregation as a possible solution for improving African American children's scholastic abilities.

Jensen juxtaposed "extreme environmental deprivation" (referring to sensory and motor restrictions of an extreme kind) with "cultural disadvantage" or deprivation. Citing research on children raised in deprived environments, such as infants in orphanages and a child confined to an attic by her deaf-mute mother, Jensen claimed that children suffering from environmental or sensory deprivation typically had depressed IQs at an early age. Following exposure to normal environmental stimulation, sensorily deprived children's IQs rose quickly and permanently. In contrast, Jensen argued, citing recent studies of school-age African American children from low-income backgrounds, culturally deprived children showed only slight initial gains in IQ after their first few months of exposure to environmental enrichment, followed by gradual declines in IQ throughout the subsequent years of schooling.[144] The net effect of his argument was to emphasize the differences between cultural and sensory deprivation. While robust experimental data proved the role of sensory deprivation in preventing normal intellectual development, Jensen argued, there was no evidence that cultural deprivation amounted to sensory deprivation or that cultural deprivation in itself could explain restricted intellectual development. Furthermore, Jensen cited studies showing that malnutrition during the prenatal and infant period impeded normal brain development. These studies, however, Jensen argued, had been carried out in countries in which hunger was endemic; in the United States, "such gross nutritional deprivation is rare." Still, citing an American study examining maternal vitamin deficiency, Jensen conceded that vitamin and mineral supplementation could be beneficial in cases where such deficiencies were proven.[145]

Hunt, a longtime proponent of compensatory education, wrote a lengthy critique of Jensen's claims. Hunt described in great detail the physiological and psychological effects of numerous experiments in sensory deprivation, spanning the analysis of retinas of rabbits raised in the dark to the study of thalami of kittens who had one eye covered for three months, as well his own recent study that examined the blink response in infants with and without colorful patterns placed over their cribs for stimulation. He argued that these works illustrated the plasticity of the nervous system, thus highlighting the role of environment in determining intellectual development.[146] Jensen retorted that Hunt was confusing cultural and sensory deprivation, arguing that disadvantaged children did not suffer from sensory deprivation in their home environment, a viewpoint held by most early education researchers at the time.[147] While Jensen distinguished between cultural disadvantage and sensory deprivation in a manner supportive of his hereditarian theory of intelligence, this distinction was the exception rather than the norm. More common was a broad, practically ecumenical interpretation of deprivation that encompassed maternal, nutritional, social, and other forms.[148]

Psychologist Jerome Kagan published a succinct four-page response in the *Harvard Educational Review* in which he argued that the theory of compensatory education had not been adequately tested. It would be nonsense, he explained, to "assume that feeding animal protein to a seriously malnourished child for three days would lead to a permanent increase in his weight and height, if after 72 hours of steak and eggs he was sent back to his malnourished environment." Similarly, after only eight weeks of summer intervention, it was impossible to conclude that compensatory education had failed. Kagan relied on the analogy between malnutrition and cultural deprivation to argue that the intervention had not been sufficiently tested.[149]

Malnutrition was not the only form of deprivation Kagan cited in his rebuttal of Jensen's hereditarian thesis. Kagan described his unpublished research findings, which documented "detailed observations of the mother child interaction" in low-income homes. Based on these observations, he argued that "lower-class children do not experience the quality of parent child interaction that occurs in the middle-class homes." While at first referring to "parents" in general, he went on to describe "lower-class mothers" as spending less time vocalizing and smiling at their infants and as not responding appropriately to their children's efforts. The absence of these experiences, Kagan argued, impeded intellectual development and led to lower test scores.[150] Kagan effectively relied on maternal deprivation theory to explain class and (implicitly) racial differences in test scores and to discredit Jensen's basic argument.

In a subsequent issue of the *Harvard Educational Review*, Martin Deutsch published a scathing critique of Jensen's essay. Deutsch, who had previously collaborated with Jensen in coediting *Social Class, Race, and Psychological Development*, dedicated to the memory of Martin Luther King Jr., criticized Jensen's work as reflecting a "consistent bias toward a racist hypothesis." Citing the "many erroneous statements, misinterpretations, and misunderstandings" in Jensen's work, Deutsch provided a comprehensive critique of Jensen's argument, citing different statistic analyses and interpretative disagreements as well as criticizing his inattention to data on deprivation.[151] Criticizing Jensen's "lack of any explanation" for "preferring" a hereditarian approach over other possible theories, Deutsch argued that Jensen had ignored important studies in the field of nutrition carried out in the United States rather than in Third World countries. These studies, Deutsch argued, proved the importance not only of maternal nutrition but even of a child's grandmother's nutrition in the child's intellectual development.[152] Sensory deprivation research provided the second part of Deutsch's critique. He referred to the work of his wife, psychologist Cynthia Deutsch, published in the volume he and Jensen had jointly edited. Her chapter had relied on key studies in the field of sensory deprivation, including Hebb's, to argue that the "slum child" is sensorily deprived.[153] Martin Deutsch believed that Cynthia Deutsch's interpretation of data from sensory deprivation experiments and her call to take into account the sensory stimulation provided by classrooms and learning materials were salient scientific evidence that Jensen had not addressed. Once again, sensory deprivation experiments were viewed as evidence of the veracity of the cultural deprivation hypothesis and were used to argue against hereditarian views of the determinants of intelligence.

African American educator William Brazziel excoriated Jensen's work as providing a basis for perpetuating segregation and strengthening theories of white intellectual supremacy.[154] In particular, he criticized Jensen for ignoring research on the effects of "brain damages wrought by malnourishment" among black children in the South, studies to which Brazziel did not refer by name. Brazziel criticized Jensen's inattention to the "deprivation axioms" made popular by researchers at the University of Chicago and called for a closer look at the "brain stunting" caused a "lack of early stimulation."[155] Brazziel argued that any strategy for addressing the racial gap on scholastic tests would ultimately have to include integrated schools free from racial and class prejudice. Citing research that found that black children in integrated schools scored closer to "white norms on achievement tests," he concluded by sardonically suggesting that these children picked up "the mysteries of Jensen's 'g-factor' through association . . . while the white children pick[ed] up the mysteries of 'soul.'"[156]

Warning that Jensen's findings would be used as an apologia for segregationists, Brazziel's rebuttal relied on studies evaluating the results of integration. Rejecting a biological theory of inherent intelligence, Brazziel highlighted "real" biological differences that resulted from the nutritional and early sensory deprivation of developing brains. For Brazziel, deprivation was the framework by which to interpret biological difference.

Jensen's approach highlighted the differences between sensory deprivation and what he termed "cultural disadvantage." In fact, Jensen continued to rely on sensory deprivation studies to argue for a hereditary component of intelligence. In a later publication, Jensen refuted the theory of "language deprivation" as an explanation for lower scholastic achievement among disadvantaged children. Some experts, he explained, argued that the use of dialect and "ungrammatical" English led to a disadvantage on tests designed to evaluate intelligence. If this were true, he argued, one would expect that African Americans would obtain their lowest scores on verbal tests and score higher on nonverbal and performance tests. Reviewing different test averages, he argued that this was not the case. African American children, regardless of socioeconomic status, attained their best results on tests evaluating verbal ability. Furthermore, Jensen argued that the "verbal deprivation hypothesis of Negro IQ deficit" would predict that the "most disadvantaged Negroes with the lowest IQ"—those living in the rural South—would show a greater deficit on verbal tests than on nonverbal tests.[157] Yet in test score statistics, the "presumably most deprived Southern Negroes" in fact performed better than their peers in the northern states. Finally, Jensen compared African American children to children born entirely deaf, which, he argued, constituted a "severe form of verbal and language deprivation." Nonhearing children attained their lowest scores on verbal portions of testing—a pattern exactly opposite to the results of African American children. Finally, Jensen argued that deaf children gradually achieved better results on tests after beginning school, eventually attaining the same results on intelligence tests as their hearing peers. In contrast, African American children who entered the school system immediately "begin to lag in linguistic and intellectual development," obtaining consistently lower results than their white peers. These arguments brought Jensen to conclude that the language deprivation theory of the "Negro-white IQ difference simply does not accord with the facts."[158] Jensen thus relied on studies of deaf children as a model of sensory deprivation to refute the language deprivation theory of the interracial achievement gap.

The debate between Jensen and prominent proponents of compensatory education demonstrates the central role of metaphors of deprivation in the nature-nurture debate. Images of malnutrition were invoked by both Jensen and his detractors, while studies of sensory deprivation in animals and in humans were presented as both supporting and rebutting the theory of cultural deprivation. Cultural deprivation, in turn, was often used interchangeably with race- and class-specific descriptions of maternal deprivation, demonstrating the significance of theories of deprivation in explaining the racial gap in test scores designed to measure intelligence and scholastic aptitude.

Conclusion

Although widely accepted as a scientific theory, cultural deprivation in fact was not a distinct field of knowledge and was based on no empirical evidence. Rather, its scientific legitimacy was derived from the better-established fields of maternal and sensory deprivation, allowing cultural deprivation theorists to provide political interpretations for seemingly neutral experimental and psychological observations. In fact, the analogies between different forms of deprivation that had become commonplace in psychological discourse by the early 1960s were also used to reframe older research in the field. In 1945, psychologist William Goldfarb published what became an often-cited comparison between children in institutions and those who received continued foster care. He concluded that institutionalized children were psychologically deprived.[159] More than thirty years later, Goldfarb claimed that he, René Spitz, David Levy, and other researchers working in the 1930s and 1940s had found strong evidence that "cultural deprivation," a term that at the time had not yet been coined, had a deleterious impact on children's growth and development.[160] Examining children's prolonged separation from their primary caregivers in settings such as hospitals and orphanages, these studies all belonged to the field of maternal deprivation. This anachronism demonstrates that by the 1970s, even leading psychologists and researchers no longer differentiated among the different forms of deprivation.

Cultural deprivation theory was not an inevitable interpretation of scientific findings but rather a politically motivated conceptual framework. Using a deprivation-based framework to view certain findings at times required considerable interpretative virtuosity. Yet this theory gained wide-spread recognition and acceptance. African Americans were often portrayed as suffering from severe environmental deficits, and their faulty home lives were blamed for their inadequate social adjustment. Antiracist and African American scholars rejected many cultural deprivation theorists' assumptions regarding the inadequacy of black families and their home lives while accepting the implicit analogies among sensory, maternal, and cultural deprivation. Ironically, Jensen, a hereditarian and racialist psychologist, uniquely rejected the merger of sensory and cultural deprivation. Scholars quibbled over the extent of deprivation, its onset, and its manifestations. Yet until the late 1960s, the framework of a deprivation-based theory was accepted across the board, with Kenneth Clark as a notable exception.

Why did researchers and governmental officials choose to view interracial and socioeconomic class differences through a framework of deficiency, highlighting what these children lacked? This approach, as Clark suggested, replaced biological inferiority with cultural deficiency, thus perpetuating Euro-American middle-class families as the scientifically sanctioned approach to child rearing. Yet unlike the essentialist biological approaches of the past, cultural deprivation led to concrete, often government-funded interventions—most famously, Project Head Start, which was designed to provide precisely the components that were seen to be lacking.

Cultural deprivation is no longer an accepted term in the discourses of American mental health and public policy. Embraced by liberal social scientists and policymakers in the 1950s and 1960s, approaches highlighting perceived damages or deficits were often deemed racist by the 1970s. What was defined as "racist" expanded rapidly in the late 1960s and early 1970s to include views that previously had been widespread, and that label was wielded as a powerful moral judgment. What had been the popular approach of racial liberals and antiracist scholars soon became seen as the purview of racial conservatives and even racists.[161] Oscar Lewis was widely identified as a liberal scholar committed to antipoverty activism. In fact, Lewis and his theory of an endemic, invisible underclass were seen as so radical that the Federal Bureau of Investigation kept tabs on his work and whereabouts.[162] Ironically, since the mid-1970s, both Lewis's "culture of poverty" theory and theories of cultural deprivation have been closely identified with the conservative agenda and held to be racist. Only recently have liberal-leaning researchers resumed addressing questions dealing with culture and poverty.[163]

Still, culture is no longer viewed as something one may or may not have, and the traditions and heritages of different populations, including minorities and persons of low socioeconomic strata, are held to be meaningful and valuable in themselves. Yet while policymakers, physicians, and educators commonly hold these positions, they often reside alongside a conceptual framework that still highlights presumed deficiencies. Educators and health professionals often see children from low-income families and culturally or linguistically diverse backgrounds as lacking in motivation, parental support, or learning habits. Current education reformers strive to shift the focus from deficits to differences.[164]

Cultural deprivation theory not only reflected deeply ingrained stereotypes of low-income and minority families but also had a long-lasting effect in reinforcing these stereotypes. Examining the roots of this deprivation-based approach and locating it within a larger discourse on deprivation provides useful insight about how this highly political theory became so widely accepted and how it acquired such a wide range of spheres of influence.

CHAPTER THREE

Targeting Deprivation
Early Enrichment and Community Action

IN 1967, journalist Fred Powledge published a short book describing the early intervention program run by psychologist Martin Deutsch at New York City's Institute for Developmental Studies (IDS). This preschool program, which had opened its doors in 1962 to African American children in Harlem, later served as a model for Project Head Start. Funded by the Anti-Defamation League, Powledge's book offered a glowing description of the program down to the smallest details. A colorful ring-stacking toy, made of movable rings of wood of decreasing diameter on an upright base, was repainted a solid yellow, Powledge explained, as part of an approach the IDS termed "isolation of stimuli." A toy that consisted of parts in both different sizes and different colors would have been overwhelming for these children; with all the rings the same color, the children could focus solely on their size.[1]

Why did the educators at the IDS believe that African American children from low-income homes would be overwhelmed by a multicolored toy? Well-meaning educators tried to provide these children, singularly described as "deprived," with what they were seen to lack. The IDS staff believed that these children had not been exposed to sufficient sensory stimulation in their homes and wanted to gradually introduce them to different colors, shapes, and sounds. Many child development experts and educators in the early 1960s shared this approach.

Cultural deprivation theory provided the scientific basis for numerous early enrichment programs in the late 1950s and early 1960s across the United States. Yet cultural deprivation theory, based on data from better-established forms of deprivation, and particularly maternal, sensory, and nutritional deprivation, lacked any robust theoretical basis. Accordingly, the intervention programs focused almost exclusively on providing sensory stimulation and individual attention as a means of compensating for the perceived sensory and maternal deprivation experienced by children from low-income homes.

76

Although many of these programs were short-lived and today are relatively obscure, at the time they were at the center of the heated debate on the role of compensatory education. Furthermore, these programs provided models for the federally funded Project Head Start.

The best-known legacy of the War on Poverty, Head Start, which now enrolls close to a million children every year, has served more than twenty-five million children (and their families) since its inception in 1965. Head Start has endured decades of political turmoil to become a pillar of American culture, maintaining bipartisan support. Four programs have particularly been credited for providing the framework and impetus for the development of Head Start.[2] The first was Bettye Caldwell and Julius Richmond's early enrichment program at Syracuse (see chapter 1), which led Richmond, a pediatrician, to be appointed as the first director of the Head Start program. The three other programs are discussed in this chapter: Susan Gray and Rupert Klaus's Early Training Project at Peabody College in Nashville and the IDS program and one run by Mobilization for Youth (MFY), both in New York City. Although all of these programs ostensibly were designed to combat "cultural deprivation," they in fact focused on preventing sensory, maternal, and nutritional deprivation. The MFY was a community action program designed to empower persons from minority ethnic backgrounds living in low-income neighborhoods. Despite the MFY's radical goals and structure, many of its interventions echoed the same language of deprivation evident in more conservative programs. When Project Head Start was established in 1965 and in the program's early years, its backers, politicians and child development experts alike, relied heavily on deprivation theory in articulating its scientific rationale and in countering the severe criticisms of the program.

The Early Training Project

The Early Training Project, an intervention program for disadvantaged preschool children, was established by Nashville psychologists Susan Gray and Rupert Klaus in 1959. Funded by the National Institute of Mental Health (NIMH), this program targeted low-income children in Murfreesboro, a town south of Nashville with a population of approximately twenty-five thousand, including many low-income African American families. The intervention, designed to offset "the progressive retardation in cognitive development and school achievement that characterizes the culturally deprived child," was carried out solely on African American children, with whom the authors believed the chances of success would be greater, though they did not elaborate why.[3] The program consisted of two components. The first was an intensive ten-week summer enrichment program that provided "typical" preschool educational experiences for low-income children, such as learning to name colors or taking turns playing with a toy. The second component consisted of weekly home sessions with a "specially trained home visitor" who would work with the children's mothers.[4] The visitors, who had studied either preschool education or social work, guided mothers in improving their parenting skills through "role-playing" in which the parents took on the role of the children and the visitors read stories or provided guidance through educational activities such as gathering colored autumn leaves.[5] Additional home interventions were designed to "foster a better understanding of the role of the Negro American in today's world." The mothers received monthly copies of *Ebony*, and the home visitors would go over the magazines with the mothers to "point out articles and pictures about successful accomplishments of Negroes."[6] The children were tested before, during, and after this two-pronged intervention, and the program was demonstrated to have lasting effects in improving poor children's scholastic achievement.[7]

Gray and Klaus presented the results of their program at a 1964 symposium, Early Experimental Deprivation and Enrichment and Later Development, chaired by Donald O. Hebb, an eminent psychologist who had pioneered early sensory deprivation experiments at McGill University. The diverse subjects included early childhood enrichment alongside research on sensory deprivation in animals.[8] When the *New York Times* described the panel, it focused mainly on Gray and Klaus's work examining "the effects of greater stimulation on the development of Negro children" from deprived backgrounds. The article also cited other scientists on the same panel who had found that kittens became quicker learners when weaned in a room with more stimulation available, while baby monkeys in "an environment barren of stimuli" were found to have abnormal mental development. The journalist made no comment regarding the difference in the methodologies used in experimental studies on animals and the preschool intervention for disadvantaged children.[9] Sensory deprivation was seen to be equally applicable in experiments carried out on laboratory animals and in preschool intervention programs.

In a 1965 article in *Child Development*, Gray and Klaus described the perceived deficiencies of the children's home lives through a unique theoretical framework they had developed. This framework examined the children's home situation in terms of "three stimulus potential and five reinforcement dimensions." This "stimulus potential" in fact referred to sensory stimulation, and the three aspects the researchers examined were the gross amount of stimulus input, its variety, and its structure. Although the children were seen to be exposed to as much "gross stimuli" as their middle-class peers, those stimuli were not sufficiently varied and unstructured and thus did not contribute to the creation of an educational environment. The authors emphasized the disorder and monotony of the sensory input available in low-income homes. The television was on all day, creating noisy but unproductive stimulation, "everybody's possessions are higgledy-piggledy and the day is not organized around such standing patterns as regular mealtimes." Thus, the children could not benefit from a clear structure of regulated environmental stimuli.[10] The mothers were occupied with "subsistence activities" and had less time to spend with their children, thus depriving them of individual attention. Rather than being educated and stimulated, Gray and Klaus lamented, these children were "often shooed out of the way of the mother at work."[11] Thus both sensory and maternal deprivation were held as major factors in the home environment of culturally deprived families. Furthermore, in addition to providing preschool experiences to the children, the intervention program included individual coaching with each mother to "develop in her more awareness of the instrumental acts involved in her child's attaining these [scholastic] aspirations."[12]

This program was widely cited as a successful example of early intervention and served as the basis for later enrichment programs. Thus, its reliance on theories of sensory and maternal deprivation is particularly significant, as is their implementation solely on a cohort of African American children.[13] Indeed, from their inception, the early intervention programs of the 1960s attempting to "combat cultural deprivation" among low-income children focused on the perceived sensory and maternal deprivation in African American families. In 1966, Gray served on the Presidential Task Force on Early Childhood Development, chaired by Joseph McVicker Hunt, which evaluated early childhood interventions, including Project Head Start. The task force, closely followed by President Lyndon Baines Johnson, produced a report recommending effective ways to provide compensatory education for disadvantaged children.[14]

That year, Gray and her colleagues reported the success of their intervention in a book published by the prestigious Columbia University Teachers College Press. Again, the authors highlighted the difficulties of these "deprived" children in performing age-appropriate learning tasks, which the authors directly attributed to inadequate home lives. For example, deprived children were described as having difficulties in distinguishing between a rabbit with symmetrical ears and one with a clearly lopsided ear. This perceived disability was seen as a direct result of the child's disorganized home life, which made it difficult if not impossible for the child to develop adequate sensory discrimination. The authors asked pointedly, "How can he see in what ways cooking pans are alike or different if the two are lying in a welter of a dozen other objects, rather than hanging side by side on hooks?"[15] The implication is clear: Disorder in the home environments of low-income families (solely African American) impeded the child's intellectual development.

In contrast, the middle-class home environment was portrayed as a natural laboratory for the child's intellectual development. The example of the skewed cooking pans clearly demonstrates gender perceptions: The inadequate kitchen, the mother's traditional realm, is metonymic with maternal care.[16] The mother's failure to keep an organized kitchen amounted to her failure to provide an adequate learning environment for her young child. This point was reiterated in the descriptions of the second component of the intervention. Staff members visited the children's homes, encouraging mothers "to become interested, or more interested, in their children." Gray and her colleagues seemed to believe that lack of maternal interest constituted a major barrier to children's intellectual development. They developed a model interaction to arouse mothers' interest in their children's learning and development. The home visitor would first ask mothers whether they were teachers. The mothers would demur, and then staff members would explain that the mothers *were* in fact teachers—their children's first teachers. After this opening, the educators would explain the significance of mothers' teaching roles, instructing them about what they should teach their preschoolers.[17] Helping mothers become involved in their children's learning was seen as a necessary part of the intervention to combat cultural deprivation.

Martin Deutsch and the IDS

Martin Deutsch's Institute for Developmental Studies was one of the most influential early intervention programs of the 1960s. Established in 1958 on the outskirts of Harlem, the institute was funded by private philanthropic foundations including the Ford Foundation and the Taconic Foundation, as well as by the Office of Economic Opportunity and the NIMH.[18] The IDS combined research with early childhood intervention programs designed to compensate for cultural disadvantage or deprivation and in 1962 began its first preschool intervention program. Four years later, the IDS became part of the New York University School of Education. Influenced by Hunt and other environmentalists, Deutsch worked to provide necessary environmental stimulation for children from home environments seen to be insufficiently stimulating.[19] A native New Yorker trained at Columbia University, Deutsch was dedicated to serving the city's disadvantaged children and was confident that socioeconomic status rather than race caused scholastic difficulties.[20]

The IDS preschool program served children from minority ethnic backgrounds, mainly African American children and a few Hispanics. Prior to 1962, the IDS staff had also evaluated white children in studies comparing children from different ethnic backgrounds matched according to socioeconomic status. Yet once the IDS shifted from being solely a research institute to developing an intervention program, it targeted primarily African American children, a decision that went unexplained. In fact, the theoretical background of the program's goals and methods refers solely to socioeconomic status, not to race. Some descriptions of the program omitted race altogether, instead highlighting the fact that it served children from low-income homes in the Harlem area.[21] While ignoring the choice of focus on African American children, Deutsch and his colleagues presumed to understand the cultural background of the families, providing what the educators perceived as race- and gender-appropriate reading material for the children's parents.

Powledge's 1967 book on the IDS opened with a detailed description of poverty's detrimental effects on the intellectual development of young children and the ensuing scholastic disadvantage. He articulated in simple terms Deutsch's theory of the role of "stimulus deprivation" in hindering the intellectual development of children raised in impoverished environments. Only one sentence of the twelve-page introduction specifically addressed race: According to Powledge, "memories of slavery" and "racial discrimination" perpetuated a "caste system" in American society.[22] Yet race was not unacknowledged. Powledge described a table with reading material for visiting parents that contained Arna Bontemps's *Story of the Negro* (1948), James Baldwin's *Go Tell It on the Mountain* (1953), and Martin Luther King Jr.'s *Strength to Love* (1963) alongside issues of *Ebony* and *Women's Day*.[23] Though these books were undoubtedly important, they also reflected what was seen as appropriate, moderate African American history for parents. No representations of the burgeoning field of black nationalism, for example, were included. The IDS staff clearly found King's *Strength to Love* more palatable and educational than Malcolm X's 1965 autobiography.

Deutsch's publications on the IDS preschool were heavily grounded in sensory deprivation research. In explaining the cause of low-income children's scholastic disadvantage, Deutsch suggested a model of sensory deprivation that referred not to the "quantity of stimulation, but rather, a restriction to a segment of the spectrum of stimulation potentially available." Thus the low-income children were seen as having been exposed not to *less* stimulation but simply to the wrong kind. "While these children have broomsticks and usually a ball, possibly a doll or a discarded kitchen pot to play with," Deutsch maintained, "they don't have the different shapes and colors and sizes to manipulate which the middle-class child has."[24] The middle-class environment contained the right playthings to provide the correct forms of stimulation. A remedy for these "major deficits in the perceptual area" would be early intervention with an emphasis on perceptual training.[25] Deutsch relied on sensory deprivation research, including psychologist Jerome Bruner's paper presented at the 1961 Harvard symposium on sensory deprivation and Hunt's book, *Intelligence and Experience,* to argue that "the experiential deprivations associated with poverty are disintegrative and subtractive from normative growth expectancies."[26]

Martin Deutsch's wife and collaborator, Cynthia Deutsch, demonstrated a similar view of the importance of sensory deprivation in her chapter, "Environment and Perception," in a volume coedited by Martin Deutsch, Irwin Katz, and Arthur Jensen. She cited at length the findings of sensory deprivation experiments on animals and on human subjects. In light of the lack of direct evidence regarding the effect of socioeconomic class on sensory perception, she argued, these experiments could be seen as relevant to early preschool interventions.[27] She described the home conditions of the "slum child" as providing "less variety of stimuli in the home" and "less verbal interaction with the child." As a result, she argued, the "slum child" arrived at school with "poorer [perceptual] discrimination performance than his middle-class counterpart." Intervention programs that could provide adequate and appropriate sensory stimulation, Deutsch maintained, could enhance the development of perceptual discrimination. She outlined the different ways in which early childhood educators could promote such a stimulating environment, modeling her recommendations on her experience at the IDS. Educators at the IDS made a point to organize beads by color

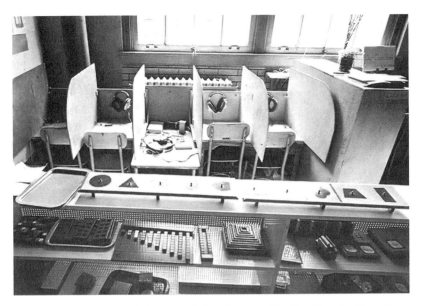

Classroom organization at the Institute for Developmental Studies. Photo by Kenneth Wittenberg. Reproduced from Fred Powledge, *To Change a Child: A Report on the Institute for Developmental Studies* (Chicago: Anti-Defamation League, 1967).

groups in clear plastic boxes "so that the color differences can be clearly seen," thus facilitating sensory stimulation.[28]

The physical organization of the classroom environment was seen as of primary importance in enhancing sensory stimulation. Publications and progress reports on the IDS invariably included detailed descriptions of how the physical environment was designed to optimize stimulation. In fact, Martin Deutsch and his IDS colleagues prepared an unpublished memorandum on "facilities for early childhood education" that included detailed measurements and architectural recommendations for designing and organizing a stimulating classroom. Windows, for example, were useful only if they provided a stimulating view of the outside world. If not, pictures and decorations were preferable; the function of letting in light and air could be achieved through "skylights and translucent wall materials" without losing "valuable wall space."[29] Deutsch's principle of "isolation of stimuli," as illustrated in the case of the all-yellow stacking toy, was evident in many of his pedagogic recommendations. Children learned colors one by one to avoid "overwhelming" them with stimulation, and they were not to be derailed by combining different shapes with different colors. A "perceptually clear and distinct room environment" helped the child focus on the learning curriculum without

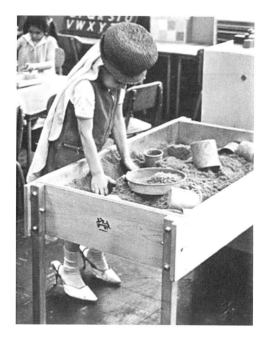

An indoor sandbox provides tactile stimulation at the Institute for Developmental Studies. Photo by Kenneth Wittenberg. Reproduced from Fred Powledge, *To Change a Child: A Report on the Institute for Developmental Studies* (Chicago: Anti-Defamation League, 1967).

"distracting him with irrelevant or diffused stimuli," as was often the case in "noisy" and cluttered home environments. A classroom sandbox provided tactile stimulation.[30]

Some of the interventions seemed to border on the comical. Deutsch argued that many of the children at the IDS did not "seem to know that people and objects have names," and some children did not even know their own names.[31] Accordingly, the teachers were instructed to address the children by name as often as possible and to display their printed names prominently throughout the classroom.[32] This gradual approach to teaching children names of people and objects was compared to "teaching standard English as a second language."[33] Books were to be straightforward and realistic; the children did not yet have a firm "perceptual and conceptual basis" that would enable them to comprehend "wildly fanciful" stories, which might be overwhelming.[34] Such prescriptions exemplified the practice of overzealously interpreting sensory deprivation research in the classroom.

The IDS received much public exposure thanks to journalist Charles Silberman. In his 1964 best-selling critique of race relations in the United States, *Crisis in Black and White*, Silberman depicted the IDS as a solution to America's most pressing problem: enabling low-income African American children to make their way in mainstream culture. Silberman also cited research by

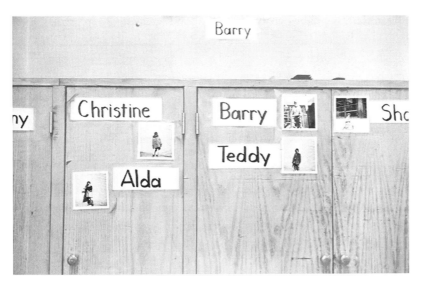

Children's names are displayed prominently at the Institute for Developmental Studies. Photo by Kenneth Wittenberg. Reproduced from Fred Powledge, *To Change a Child: A Report on the Institute for Developmental Studies* (Chicago: Anti-Defamation League, 1967).

Joseph McVicker Hunt and "culture of poverty" anthropologist Oscar Lewis. Steeped in these studies, Silberman articulated his conclusions in a language rife with deprivation metaphors.[35] The "intellectual and sensory poverty" of the African American child's environment was a significant source of developmental disadvantage. Like many before him, Silberman argued that low-income homes were in effect "non-verbal." Adults spoke in monosyllables, and children there never heard "several sentences spoken consecutively."[36] Silberman consequently concluded that "to reverse the effects of a starved environment—to provide the sensory and verbal and visual stimuli that are necessary for future learning," school should begin as early as age three.[37]

Silberman's laudatory review of Deutsch's work reverberated among policymakers. As historian Maris Vinovskis has shown, politicians cited an article Silberman published in *Harper's Magazine* in their debates over early childhood education. Speaking to members of the House Subcommittee on the War on Poverty Program, Pennsylvania Democrat William S. Moorhead called on his colleagues to "give careful consideration to Mr. Silberman's proposals" for developing large-scale early intervention programs. Furthermore, educators who had previously focused only on grade-school education started to refer to early preschool intervention in the months following the publication of Silberman's article.[38] Thus, Silberman had an important role in shifting public debate over childhood education from grade school to the toddler and preschool years. He also contributed to reifying the view of minorities and low-income families as suffering from a form of sensory deprivation. In a recursive manner, *Crisis in Black and White* later served as a textbook in an IDS training program that was designed to educate teachers "in Negro history and the problems of modern day ghetto life."[39]

The IDS, the MFY, and the Ford Foundation

White liberal experts did not see this deprivation-based approach as condescending or judgmental toward the African American community. Somewhat surprisingly, Deutsch's research and the IDS intervention found a receptive audience among activists in MFY, an influential New York community action program.

The MFY was conceived in 1957 as a juvenile delinquency prevention program by the Henry Street Settlement, a nonprofit social service agency that operated on the Lower East Side, an area with a high Latino and African American population. In the early 1950s, juvenile delinquency emerged as a topic of great concern and anxiety for the American public and was quickly taken up by politicians and scientific experts. Much of the debate centered on the loss of parental authority and the corrupting influence of mass culture, such as comic books and radio programs. Psychiatrists were called upon to weigh in on the causes and possible solutions to the "epidemic" of juvenile delinquency. Psychiatrist Fredric Wertham famously warned against comic books' "seduction of the innocent," and mental health experts were seen as the authority to explain the causes of juvenile misbehavior and criminality.[40] Yet despite public alarm at the rising number of youth offenders committing violent crimes, stricter punishments were not seen as the solution, as later became the case. Rather, policymakers emphasized understanding the causes of juvenile delinquency and developing effective preventative programs.[41] Recent scholarship has suggested that this approach reflected the racial makeup of the offenders. By the late 1950s, crime had increasingly become associated with African American and Latino male perpetrators, a development that led to demands by politicians and the American public for a "crackdown" on crime and stricter sentencing.[42] Until the mid-1950s, however, psychologically oriented theories of juvenile crime abounded, many of which found fault with the young white offenders' parents. As one sociologist told *Newsweek* in 1954, referring to broken homes and inattentive parents, "there doesn't seem to be enough love to go around any more."[43] In *West Side Story*, which premiered on Broadway in 1957, Action, the leader of the all-white gang, the Jets, quips, "I'm depraved on account I'm deprived," in response to his friend who, impersonating a judge, had pronounced, "This child is depraved on account he ain't had a normal home."[44] Deprivation in this case meant maternal, rather than cultural deprivation. Indeed throughout the 1950s, when theories of deprivation were used to explain the rise of juvenile delinquency, they referred solely to maternal deprivation and were used to describe offenders from Euro-American backgrounds.

By the late 1950s, when the media increasingly reported stories of offenses committed by African American and Latino males, and a New York City judge suggested discouraging migration of minorities into the city to prevent the rise of delinquency, both African American and liberal social action programs recognized the wisdom of high-visibility programs targeting juvenile delinquency in minority communities.[45] As the focus shifted to minorities in the early 1960s, cultural deprivation received new emphasis as a cause of juvenile delinquency. In the previous decades, the NIMH had supported numerous projects focusing on juvenile delinquency, including the Judge Baker Clinic in Boston, which emphasized the personal, intrapsychic aspects of delinquency. Influenced by research in social psychology and urban studies, the NIMH changed its funding priorities, seeking comprehensive programs that offered structural solutions to the problem of delinquency.[46]

The MFY fit within this new research agenda. Although one MFY research proposal was rejected by the NIMH in 1958, organizers received clear instructions for how to prepare a successful second proposal. The NIMH required that the proposal demonstrate that the Lower East Side community was actively involved in the project and specified that the proposal must contain both research and evaluation components. Furthermore, the NIMH dictated that the MFY project join forces with what were termed "indigenous" residents (the target population of the intervention) as well as with social scientists. The NIMH approved a revised research proposal in 1961, the year the MFY officially began its action. It received additional funding from the Ford Foundation and the President's Committee on Juvenile Delinquency.[47]

The theoretical orientation of the revised proposal was based on "opportunity theory."[48] First articulated by sociologists Lloyd Ohlin and Richard Cloward, consultants for the Ford Foundation, and published in their influential book, *Delinquency and Opportunity* (1960), this theory argued that opportunities for advancement were unevenly distributed among social strata.

Ohlin and Cloward claimed that a lack of legitimate opportunities for social advancement led youth to choose illegitimate options for advancement and self-empowerment, such as criminal behavior. This theory profoundly influenced perceptions of criminality and provided the intellectual framework for a number of influential antidelinquency intervention programs, including the MFY.[49] The MFY was designed to provide youth with legitimate opportunities, thereby creating a framework for addressing problems of juvenile delinquency and poverty in a population composed mainly of low-income persons of color.

The Ford Foundation, at the time the nation's largest and most influential philanthropic organization and a major funder of the IDS, provided substantial money for the MFY.[50] The Ford Foundation's educational program clearly adopted a deprivation-based approach to early childhood education, as is evidenced both by its funding priorities and choices and by a number of publications and reports prepared by the foundation's director of education and research, Marjorie Martus. Her report, "The Special Case of the Young Disadvantaged Child," cited experimental research on sensory deprivation as a potential cause for scholastic disadvantage among low-income children while arguing that the "development of learning abilities is of course intimately related to personal interaction, particularly the mother-child relationship." She warned that research had shown that learning difficulties might arise from "the absence of a warm intimate relationship between mother and child."[51] Reviewing the work of Martin and Cynthia Deutsch as an important contribution to describing the "specific areas of deficiency" in low-income children, Martus clearly portrayed disadvantaged children as suffering from both sensory and maternal deprivation.[52] Similarly, in a 1965 report on early childhood education, Martus surveyed sensory deprivation research carried out on animals, including the early Hebb experiments, and observational studies conducted on institutionalized infants. She thus tied together research on sensory and maternal deprivation to provide the scientific rationale for the national interest in early preschool enrichment.[53]

Martus concurred with prevailing views that highlighted the detrimental effects of perceived sensory and maternal deprivation among children from low-income homes. Yet beyond Martus's individual perceptions of disadvantaged children, as director of educational programs at the Ford Foundation, she was responsible for recommending what programs would receive the foundation's support. Her view of children from low-income families as suffering from maternal and sensory deprivation thus perpetuated the influential role of theories of deprivation in early childhood education.

The MFY's educational programs, ostensibly based on Cloward's opportunity theory, which highlighted community involvement, and funded by the Ford Foundation, were in fact entrenched in theories of deprivation and compensation. Theories of deprivation—sensory, maternal and cultural—framed how the target population of these intervention programs was viewed and which interventions were seen as necessary. In fact, in 1962, the MFY's director, George Brager, suggested that "multi-problem" families might be more accurately described as "multi-deprived." Echoing the sensory-deprivation-based view of low-income homes, Brager argued that any program developed would need to take into account those features of low-income home life that hampered children's success in school—lack of intellectual stimulation, crowded homes, and noise and disorder. These characteristics were identical to those cited by cultural deprivation theorists at the time.[54]

The MFY Proposal: Community Action or Deprivation Compensation?

The MFY's 1961 revised proposal to the NIMH was titled *A Proposal for the Prevention and Control of Delinquency by Expanding Opportunities.*[55] The program's stated goals included empowering a disenfranchised population through community action and providing normative opportunities for individual advancement that would replace the need for delinquent behavior. These two characteristics of the proposal—the reliance on opportunity theory and the focus on community empowerment—reflected the changes the NIMH had required to approve funding and were not readily accepted by many of those involved both in the Henry Street Settlement organization and in the newly hired MFY administration. Yet, as Richard Cloward later explained, "money was the glue that held these competing factions together."[56]

The proposal highlighted the importance of "indigenous" participation, a term used throughout the 1960s, although its meanings were not always consistent. Primarily, it referred to the involvement of the individuals targeted by the intervention in its design and practice. Yet the term was used to describe a wide spectrum of involvement, from being solely the consumers of the intervention or subjects in a social science experiment to guides or interpreters who served as liaisons between the professional staff and the community. In any case, they remained outside the loci of power and in-fluence.[57] Furthermore, the MFY staff's definition of "indigenous" changed over time.[58] At first only a small number of poor residents were involved in marginal positions, but when community members, the professional staff, and funding agencies pressured for more extensive indigenous participation, the term became a filler/surrogate for race and ethnicity. In response to these demands for further democratization and community involvement, Latino and African American experts were recruited. Thus, as sociologist Joseph Helfgot has argued, the "poor were symbolically represented through minor-ity group elites" without jeopardizing the privileged role accorded to expert knowledge.[59] Yet despite its haziness, the concept of indigenous participation was a significant part of the MFY ideology and served as an inspiration for the War on Poverty's principle of "maximum feasible participation" of the poor in federally funded antipoverty programs.[60]

Alongside the focus on community action and the involvement of "in-digenous" residents, the proposal also relied on a deprivation-based inter-pretation of the needs and challenges of the program's target community.[61] Throughout the proposal, the MFY staff used deprivation metaphors to ex-plain the rationale for their proposed interventions. For example, scholastic disadvantage in children from low-income homes was seen as caused by a lack of stimulation and skills. The authors argued that "the deprived occu-pational and economic circumstances of lower-class households provide children with little intellectual stimulation, facility in manipulating abstract symbols and language, or other skills in communication."[62] This image of a "deprived lower-class household" was based on a perceived lack of both sensory stimulation and parental involvement. Economic circumstances re-sulted in a meager household with few educational objects; parents' long working hours and scanty educational background created a lack of appro-priate parental stimulation. This deprived home environment, in turn, was cited as "handicapping" these children in their social competition with their middle-class counterparts. Such "handicaps" further limited opportunities for advancement and thus perpetuated delinquency, as "systems of social stratification generate delinquent behavior by restricting opportunities."[63]

The MFY's Division of Educational Opportunities was responsible for educational intervention at all age levels, from early preschool to adult. These different educational programs sought not only to provide children from low-income and minority homes with equal educational opportunities, primarily by improving the level of the schools serving the neighborhood's children, but also to assist teachers and schools in accounting for the "class and ethnic background of the child." The MFY proposal criticized the middle-class orientation of typical school curricula and highlighted the need for teachers to transmit a "sense of appreciation of all peoples, whatever their occupation, ethnic background, class status."[64] Furthermore, the proposal called for local residents' involvement in decision making and for the establishment of parent-school programs to further integrate parents into their children's learning experiences. This approach illustrates the community action aspect of the MFY proposal, and its attempt to democratize inner-city education.

Yet the same passage also reflected the program's deprivation-based approach. School administrators and teachers needed to familiarize themselves with the homes of their students, not simply to learn more about the students' backgrounds but also to witness firsthand their deprived circumstances. Family structure was faulted for the lack of educational opportunities available for low-income children: "The need to concentrate upon bare economic survival severely limits the amount of attention parents can allocate to the 'non-essential' activity of stimulating their children's intellectual growth or planning their education future." In low-income homes, the MFY staff argued, "intellectual stimulation in the form of books, recordings, trips, and the like is lacking . . . for purely economic reasons if not for others as well." Furthermore, program officials maintained that as a consequence of "cultural deprivation, lower-class children require special attention in school," thus in effect blurring any distinction between the terms "cultural deprivation" and "lower class."[65]

The "deprived" home conditions of low-income families provided the impetus for programs designed to help teachers "understand the effect of the home upon school performance" and thus enable them to shape "the intellectual and social milieu of the classroom" according to the children's needs.[66] Although the MFY proposal criticized the quality of education available for schoolchildren in the target population, the main focus of the proposed interventions was the perceived incompatibility of teaching methods and educational content for low-income and minority children, for whom middle-class culture was seen as foreign. Accordingly, familiarizing teachers with their students' deprived home environments was seen as an important step in improving the level of education provided. Although the race and socioeconomic background of the MFY teachers was never mentioned, it seemed obvious to the researchers that the teachers would come from a different cultural background from that of their students.[67]

Citing Martin Deutsch's IDS work, the MFY proposal argued that many "culturally starved" youngsters had difficulties in primary school and traced these difficulties to the lack of stimulation in the homes of low-income minority children.[68] The MFY proposal suggested remedying this problem through an early enrichment program designed to provide the children with the experiences they lacked. This program, "geared especially to alleviating the verbal and cognitive deficiencies that underlie retardation in basic school skills," highlighted activities designed to develop "cognitive and sensory motor skills." One of its main goals was to provide "a learning environment not usually available to the child in a low socio economic area."[69]

Cooperation between the MFY and the IDS

The surprising cooperation between Martin Deutsch's IDS work and the MFY program demonstrates the MFY's entrenchment in deprivation theory. In 1963, the MFY's Educational Division contracted the IDS to develop a program of "therapeutic curricula" designed to promote first-grade readiness. MFY educators had long been interested in Deutsch's work, citing his findings in the 1961 MFY proposal as evidence for the necessity of early preschool intervention.[70] This acceptance of the IDS's theoretical approach and pedagogical methods may have also been influenced by the fact that the two organizations shared a benefactor—the Ford Foundation. Thus, the 1963 decision to contract the IDS to provide early preschool intervention further reinforced the deprivation-based approach previously evident in the MFY's educational programs.

In subsequent reports, the MFY's education program directors reiterated their belief in early enrichment as a means to "forestall later retardation and frustration."[71] Abraham J. Tannenbaum, the MFY's coordinator of education programs, was a professor of education at Columbia University who had previously worked as a teacher in a Brooklyn public school.[72] In 1965, explaining the MFY's emphasis on environmental stimulation, Tannenbaum argued that it was "well known that children from socially disadvantaged environments show deficiencies in motor development, visual perception and auditory stimulation."[73] By 1966, Tannenbaum's description of the rationale for the MFY's educational programs was even more enmeshed in sensory stimulation terminology. While there "may be a congenital basis for sensory-motor dysfunction" that led to the "deficiencies in motor development, visual perception and auditory discrimination" seen in children from disadvantaged backgrounds, Tannenbaum argued, early enrichment could still be useful in reversing this deficit.[74] This statement is remarkable because Tannenbaum referred to a possible hereditary component in the perceived deficits in low-income children's development. Although he continued to advocate on behalf of early intervention, Tannenbaum's views differed significantly from those of most proponents of early enrichment, who favored an environmentally determined view of both intelligence and psychological development. According to Tannenbaum, the MFY's educational program was designed to test the benefits of early enrichment by providing "general practice in physical coordination and balance, eye movement exercises, guided experiences in forming perceptions and developmental activities to sharpen visual memory."[75] Thus the MFY's educational programs were not only based on a perception of sensory deprivation but also coordinated by someone who accepted a possible genetic explanation for low scholastic achievement for children from low-income backgrounds.

In 1966, the MFY board of directors authorized a proposal to develop a "laboratory preschool in an urban depressed area."[76] Prepared by the MFY educational staff, the proposal was based on the assumption that lower-income children were "handicapped by a home environment." Citing the works of Deutsch and Hunt, the proposal maintained that the "deficits of the socially disadvantaged child are thought to result from inadequate experience in a variety of tasks, oversimplification of his world and little complexity in his daily life."[77] Thus, despite the community action approach publicly presented as the MFY's rationale, the educational programs were clearly based on a deprivation-based view of the needs and abilities of children from low-income, minority homes.

STAR: Between Community Action and the Deprivation Discourse

In 1965, the MFY Division of Educational Opportunities developed an early reading readiness program, Supplementary Teaching Assistance in Reading (STAR), that epitomized the tension between the MFY's proclaimed goals and theoretical basis and the prevailing discourse on deprivation. STAR, first implemented in the 1965–66 school year, was designed to train parents to assist their children in making early steps to reading. It relied on parent training by "indigenous" nonprofessional adults who lived in the program's target area and who themselves received training so that they could educate parents. According to a report Tannenbaum prepared in July 1967, this approach was not simply a way to "fill teaching positions with any available warm bodies" but was part of a conscious attempt to involve nonprofessional residents in the program.[78] The use of nonprofessionals and "indigenous involvement" were important ideological aspects of community involvement in the MFY's programs.[79] Furthermore, the program was designed to empower parents by teaching them how to teach their children, thus transforming their homes into sites of learning. Other interventions targeting low-income children, in contrast, viewed the removal of children from their home environments as therapeutic in itself.

Yet alongside this activist community involvement approach was a deprivation-based approach that found fault both with low-income children's home environments and with their mothers. Citing studies of infants raised in "foundling homes" that "revealed that poor mothering practices can inhibit healthy mental development," Tannenbaum suggested that the "early deprivation in the slum family environment" was accountable for later scholastic disadvantage. Yet again, maternal deprivation was seen as part of cultural deprivation, and studies on institutionalized infants were seen as relevant to understanding the family dynamics in low-income homes. Through the employment of nonprofessional teaching aides, Tannenbaum explained, educators would be able "to gain access" to homes earlier than other preschool interventions could. This tactic would "breathe new meaning into early intervention." Thus the use of nonprofessionals was designed to enable professionals to permeate and alter faulty home environments as early as possible. This intervention sought to offset the "deleterious effects of minimal succorant care in infancy, provide an environment of optimum cognitive stimulation . . . and build the young child's experiential background."[80] Tannenbaum did not distinguish between maternal and sensory deprivation and perceived maternal care and sensory stimulation as both critical for normal development and lacking in low-income homes. Accordingly, STAR was designed to counter the negative effects of both forms of deprivation. To summarize, STAR was based on a discourse of social activism that strove for maximum community involvement alongside a deprivation-based approach targeting maternal and sensory deprivation.

The same images of deprivation invoked in Tannenbaum's description of STAR also figured, almost verbatim, in the MFY's fundraising efforts. Herbert

Goldsmith, director of the MFY Division of Educational Opportunities, had worked as a teacher before receiving his doctorate in education from New York University. Dedicated to struggles for social justice, Goldsmith had served as vice president of the U.S. National Student Association and later became a leader in the Congress of Racial Equality.[81] Goldsmith invoked both sensory and maternal deprivation in his April 1967 letter requesting funding for the 1967–68 school year from the Taconic Foundation, a philanthropic organization dedicated to fighting racial and social inequities.

Goldsmith proposed a three-stage preschool program that would follow mothers and their children from pregnancy until first grade. The first stage consisted of a "paranatal care and training program" targeting expectant mothers and their young infants, followed by a "school orientation" program for preschool children and finally STAR to promote reading readiness. The school orientation program was designed to "enable slum parents" to better understand the "structure and function of public education in the community," thus helping them to create a more "positive orientation toward learning" in their homes and thus participate in the "ultimate educational goals of the school."[82] The earliest-stage training program was still being planned, but it would provide "guidelines for designing clear-cut sequential mother-infant activities." Using the same terminology Tannenbaum used four months later in his first STAR report, the program's goals were "1) to avoid the delecterious [*sic*] effects of minimal succorant care in infancy 2) to provide an environment of optimum cognitive stimulation at the earliest stages in life and 3) to build the young child's experiential background in preparation for learning." Citing the early descriptions of maternal deprivation by psychoanalyst René Spitz and others, Goldsmith argued that research on maternal deprivation had demonstrated that "the derogating effects of poor mothering practices are long-lasting" and that certain forms of parental behavior could inhibit healthy development. For the "slum child," therefore, early intervention might be critical. Copies of this letter were sent to the MFY's top officials, including Bertram Beck and John Niemeyer. Sharing both substance and terminology with Tannenbaum's unpublished report on STAR, the letter demonstrates that theories of sensory and maternal deprivation were well accepted by the MFY's education experts. These assumptions were also reiterated in an undated MFY report proposing a "School Orientation Program for Parents."[83] As late as 1967, by which time criticism of deprivation theory had already begun to appear, the use of sensory and maternal deprivation terminology was not seen as problematic or controversial. Early the following year, Tannenbaum published an evaluation of STAR based on the 1967 report he had prepared for the MFY. The article, which appeared in the *Teachers College Record*, included the same descriptions of the program's goals: to "head off the deleterious effects of minimal succorant care in infancy, provide an environment of optimum cognitive stimulation at the earliest stages in life, and build the young child's experiential background in preparation for learning."[84]

The MFY: A Radical Program

In the mid-1960s, the MFY came under attack. At a time when community action programs were blamed for inciting strikes, pickets, and other forms of social protest, the MFY was accused of spreading dissent and leading to social instability.[85] In the early 1960s, the MFY had backed highly controversial social struggles. For instance, it supported local leaders who sought to establish civilian review boards that would investigate allegations of police misconduct. In 1963, the MFY offered support and organizational assistance when residents challenged landlords and housing agencies by withholding rent until building violations were addressed.[86]

Critics on the political right saw these and other MFY community action programs as subversive. At the same time, liberal social workers and activists worried that the MFY would tarnish their reputation by being too radical.[87] In 1964, the MFY became the subject of an investigation that included FBI undercover agents and wiretapping in an attempt to expose what was portrayed in the popular media—particularly in the conservative *New York Daily News*—as a communist nest.[88] The investigation, supervised by New York's attorney general, ended in early 1965 when the program was cleared of all charges. The episode nonetheless tainted the public's view of the program and contributed to a decline in its support.[89] At the time, observers considered the MFY a very radical program, designed to empower and mobilize the community it served. Yet much of its educational approach was based on long-accepted theories of deprivation and compensation.

HARYOU

While the MFY was designed mainly by white liberals, Harlem Youth Opportunities Unlimited (HARYOU) was a well-publicized community action program led by and for African Americans. The organization was conceived as a protest against "social work colonialism." According to Kenneth Clark,

HARYOU arose as a reaction to New York City's 1961 decision to hire the Jewish Board of Guardians to provide psychiatric care to youth in Harlem, without involving any local agencies.[90] Relations between African Americans and Jews in New York City were fraught, and the decision to bring in experts from outside the Harlem community caused considerable dissent. In 1976, Clark candidly recalled that he had been "furious on racial or ethnic grounds," objecting to the reliance on Jewish benefactors he ironically termed "Lady Bountifuls."[91] Clark and his colleagues decided to organize a program that stressed the empowerment of the African American population and viewed white racism as one of the main factors in the disenfranchisement of this population. Having learned of the government funding the MFY received, HARYOU organizers were determined to obtain money for a program for and by the African American community.

The program was based on a theory of redistribution of power, addressing the racial oppression and political disenfranchisement the residents of Harlem suffered. Noel Cazenave has summarized the fundamental difference between the two programs: While the MFY relied on opportunity theory, HARYOU was based on a theory of power.[92] HARYOU emphasized the role white racism played in the creation of economic disparities and envisioned a massive community reorganization leading to local empowerment.[93] In their project proposal, *Youth in the Ghetto: A Study of the Consequences of Powerlessness and a Blueprint for Change*, HARYOU planners addressed the main problems of the ghetto, including education, employment, and delinquency. The political goals of this program shaped its perception of the debate on deprivation. It focused primarily on providing early educational intervention, job training, and community programs for youth in an effort to fundamentally change race relations. For example, the employment programs took pride in the fact that their vocational counselors would never recommend that advisees take marginal jobs below their personal potential just because these jobs were currently available. The comprehensive employment program was "geared toward revamping the various systems" that led to the underemployment of African Americans and the devaluing of their education. This program included not only job training but also "agitation and pressure for expanded opportunities for Negroes" by urging employers to hire HARYOU trainees.[94]

In the proposal's chapter on education, the authors outlined the debate over cultural deprivation and what they termed "the controversy of underachievement." This "controversy" centered on the question of whether Harlem students performed poorly in school because of deficits in their home environment or because of the low level of teaching and the lack of funding that characterized the neighborhood schools. The HARYOU planners summarized current theories regarding the causes of scholastic disadvantage, which highlighted the role of meager, unstimulating home environments without criticizing deprivation-based presuppositions or methodology. They cited one unreferenced description of a child who could distinguish only three colors when he entered kindergarten, a situation the authors explained as resulting from the fact that he had "simply never had the experiences which lead to color recognition."[95] They did not reject these descriptions of children growing up in unstimulating homes, implicitly accepting the argument made by Martin Deutsch and other like-minded researchers that the "low-income, minority-group child enters school without certain of the experiences and skill of the middle-class child." Yet they disagreed with the conclusion that this difference in early childhood experiences provided sufficient explanation for lower scholastic achievement. Instead, the HARYOU planners suggested that school administrators, aware of the research findings of Deutsch and other proponents of cultural deprivation theory, expected less from low-income, minority children. The result was a classroom atmosphere not conducive to academic progress. Examining statistical data indicating distinct deterioration in school achievement between the third and sixth grades, HARYOU's founders concluded that the main barriers to learning were located in the schools serving low-income and minority children rather than in their home environments. Thus, while children might reach school with differing levels of experience, skills, and attitudes, these differences, HARYOU educators argued, had not been demonstrated to constitute a permanent barrier to learning.[96] The HARYOU proposal's view of the cause of scholastic disadvantage among low-income minority children demonstrates that deprivation theory was not the inevitable conclusion of examining class and race disparities in scholastic achievement. Rather, their approach reflected the political orientations of the educators or researchers evaluating the data. While white liberal educators favored deprivation-based interpretations to explain scholastic disadvantage, African American educators viewed the same data as evidence for the faulty education children received in underfunded schools. HARYOU educators saw deprivation theory as compounding this problem by negatively influencing teachers' assumptions regarding their students' abilities.

Head Start

Project Head Start, administered by the newly established Office of Economic Opportunity (OEO), was first announced in May 1965 as an eight-week summer program. Later converted to a yearlong intervention, Head Start was designed to provide preschool-age children with experiences and training perceived to be lacking in their impoverished homes and to offset the negative effects of deprivation.[97] Project Head Start garnered much public interest and positive media coverage and in its first summer served more than half a million children.[98]

In its early years, Head Start was an eclectic network of programs that had successfully competed for federal funding.[99] As historian Maris Vinovskis has compellingly argued, Head Start was set up with the dangerous combination of great haste and inadequate budget. While Deutsch and other child development experts had estimated a budget of $1,000 per child for an eight-week summer program, the official budget allotted $180 per child. To quickly create a relatively low-budget large-scale federal program, applications openly acknowledged as of dubious quality were approved.[100] Furthermore, Project Head Start had no set curricula, educational requirements, or even clear educational goals. Thus, the programs differed greatly in educational approach and quality, and it is impossible to refer to Head Start as a monolithic early intervention program. Both the debate over Head Start's rationale and creation and the controversy surrounding early evaluations of its effectiveness were couched in deprivation terminology and reflected the merging of nutritional, sensory, and maternal deprivation theories.

Early Head Start and Deprivation

The first Head Start programs attempted to provide comprehensive care, offering educational enrichment, nutritional supplementation, and preventive medical and dental care.[101] The discourse of deprivation is abundantly evident in the early descriptions of the program. A letter to pediatric mental health experts inviting submissions for developing local Head Start programs defined the program's goal as helping children overcome "the obvious deficiencies imposed on them by poverty."[102]

While the official rationale for the program was the prevention of cultural deprivation, two distinct forms of deprivation—nutritional and sensory—

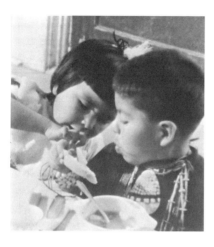

Mealtime at Project Head Start.
Reproduced from Luise K. Addiss,
Jenny Is a Good Thing (Washington,
D.C.: U.S. Department of Health,
Education, and Welfare, 1969).

figured in the early discourse.[103] A "health component" was mandatory to
obtain Head Start funding for a early intervention programs. Screening for
and preventing nutritional deficiencies were seen as having a pivotal role in
the program, a component that garnered interest from the National Vitamin Foundation and other groups involved in preventing nutritional deficiencies.[104] Participating children were screened for iron deficiency anemia
and other dietary deficiency diseases, and the intervention's goals included
changing nutritional habits through parent education.[105] Head Start pioneer
psychologist Edward Zigler recalled how nutritionists zealously labored to
change the dietary habits of low-income children and their families. In contrast, Zigler realized at the time, Project Head Start had not hired professionals with a primary specialization in children's mental health.[106] In fact, some
senior pediatricians questioned the benefits of employing mental health
professionals at all, doubting the importance of a psychiatric perspective in
what seemed to be a medical and educational endeavor.[107] While the role
of mental health experts in the program was vague, nutritional experts and
their screening and intervention programs enjoyed much prestige. Head Start
compiled cookbooks and involved children's families in culinary events, celebrating holidays with the traditional dishes of different cultures.[108] One
nutritionist who supervised two dozen Head Start centers planned Cinco de
Mayo menus for preschools that served primarily African American communities. Newspapers reprinted Head Start recipes and informed their readers
of Head Start nutritional events, including educational conferences organized for the general public.[109] Actor Burt Lancaster narrated an Academy
Award–nominated short 1969 documentary on the educational importance

of diverse culinary experiences in Head Start programs. The film was distributed among Head Start educators, accompanied by a booklet to guide discussion of the subject.[110]

The parallels among different forms of deprivation were openly acknowledged in media accounts of the Head Start nutritional programs. One article described participating children as "deprived nutritionally as well as socially," reversing the order child development experts had originally envisioned. Another extolled how "extra helpings of affection and attention go along with extra helpings of food."[111] Images of nutritional deprivation profoundly shaped how the public viewed Head Start's goals.

Head Start was committed to the prevention of sensory deprivation early in life. An OEO statement described Head Start's mission as ensuring that "no young child shall lack the environmental stimulation and opportunity which will make it possible for him to fulfill the complete range of his developmental capacities."[112] Another OEO document claimed that low-income children suffered from "clearly observable deficiencies in processes that lay the foundation for a pattern of failure—and thus a pattern of poverty—throughout the child's entire life."[113] Head Start was lauded as countering the lack of environmental stimulation—tantamount to sensory deprivation—that limited children's intellectual potential.

The First Lady, Lady Bird Johnson, was an enthusiastic supporter of early childhood intervention programs and the honorary chair of Project Head Start. At an early 1965 event announcing the program's establishment, she described the plight of children from low-income homes. Some of the children targeted by this program, she claimed, "don't even know a hundred words, because they have not heard a hundred words"; they had never seen a book or held a flower; some of them did not know their names, which their parents had failed to teach them.[114] Today, these clearly erroneous perceptions of children from low-income and minority backgrounds seem misguided, even comical. At the time, however, the First Lady and her listeners shared a negative perception of the meager environment available in low-income homes that severely restricted young children's intellectual development. Furthermore, these statements highlight the widespread acceptance of a close relationship between what was seen or heard—perceptual stimulation or experience—and the child's intellectual development. Similarly, a pediatrician offered Julius Richmond his support and assistance in Project Head Start, lamenting how "literally thousands of children have never seen a piece of paper, a book, a crayon; they have never heard a song except for what comes

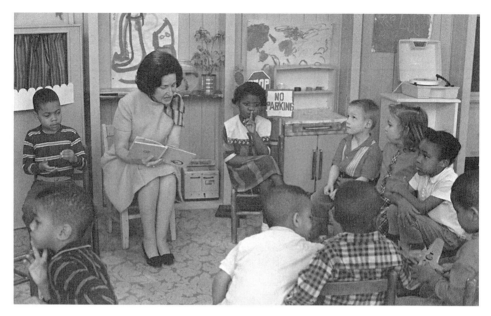

Lady Bird Johnson visits a Head Start classroom, 1968. Photo by Robert Knudsen.
Courtesy of Lyndon Baines Johnson Library and Museum, Austin, Texas.

over the radio; they have never seen pictures; they have never been stimulated in any way."[115] The views expressed by the First Lady and this pediatrician reflected prevailing perceptions. Professionals and laypersons alike shared a stereotypical view of a total lack of stimulation in low-income homes. Head Start was hailed as the panacea for this problem.

These deprivation-based perceptions were also shared by the professionals who had conceptualized, designed, and helped establish Project Head Start. Correspondence between psychologist Joseph McVicker Hunt and Julius Richmond clearly demonstrated how both psychologists and pediatricians were deeply invested in the deprivation discourse. In May 1965, Richmond invited Hunt to serve as a consultant to Head Start's "Evaluation Unit."[116] Hunt agreed to take on the task, despite his busy schedule, since he had "actively advocated enriching pre-school experience as a way of counteracting cultural deprivation." Yet he believed that Head Start was too late and too short an intervention to prevent the detrimental effects of poverty, suggesting instead a year-round, full-day enrichment program that would start when the child first started walking. At that point, "poverty gets in its lick," and the same environment that had previously provided adequate stimulation for young infant development was, according to Hunt, depriving for a toddler.

Although he had long been convinced that the preschool experience "could be a successful antidote for cultural deprivation," Hunt questioned whether Head Start could effectively achieve this goal.[117] Richmond admitted that he would have preferred to work with far younger infants and children to counter the environmental deprivation they experienced at home. However, he cautioned, in "dealing with public policy one . . . must start with a program that has acceptability." The American public was not yet ready to accept the idea of infants being separated from their mothers and placed in communal child rearing programs that reeked of socialism. Richmond added that even if Head Start did not lead to "measurable changes in the psycho-social development of the children," at least it would be effective in terms of health and nutrition.[118]

Many mid- to late 1960s publications on Head Start relied extensively on sensory deprivation research. Descriptions of laboratory sensory deprivation experiments were followed by descriptions of cultural deprivation. The authors of one article, all of whom were education specialists, described the New Nursery School they had established in 1963 in Colorado. The program, dedicated to providing an enriching and stimulating environment, served primarily Latino children. Head Start awarded the program federal funding, and beginning in 1966, the New Nursery School served as a Head Start teacher training center.[119] To explain the importance of environmental stimulation, the authors cited an experiment that had been published in *American Psychology* that found that environmental enrichment led to an increase in the weight of the cerebral cortex in rats.[120] The authors then presented anecdotal accounts of children raised in extreme states of sensory deprivation, including cases of feral children. They argued that mounting evidence showed that the same effect of sensory deprivation could be observed "in environmentally deprived children whether they come from the slums of city or from the rural country side."[121] Hence, sensory deprivation research lent scientific authority to speculation regarding "environmental" deprivation in a procession from animal experiments to severe sensory deprivation to environmental deficits among poor children. Deprived children's "drab" home environments were depicted as glum and gray: "The unpainted exterior of his house blends with the dirt yard. His mother's concern is not that the table setting should be color-coordinated and the food provide a contrast pleasing to the eye. Her concern is that there is food on the table." In middle-class homes, by contrast, children's bright environments enabled them to contrast colors and learn the names of the many available objects.[122]

This essay was published in the second volume of a trilogy edited by educator Jerome Hellmuth that included contributions by well-known figures such as white psychologist Arthur Jensen, African American psychologist Edmund Gordon, and Sargent Shriver, director of the OEO. The essay, whose authors were dedicated to improving the education of minority children, was not unique in its approach: Many articles that addressed the scientific rationale for Head Start cited findings from sensory deprivation research. In fact, the lead author, Glendon Nimnicht, who later received the first Kellogg's Child Development Award, and his wife, also an educator, later traveled to her native Colombia to head a community-based education program.[123] Although the New Nursery School justified its pedagogic approach with an at best questionable reliance on sensory deprivation theory, that does not mean that the program lacked educational value or the potential to empower and inform young children. Rather, antiracist educators dedicated to empowering minority and low-income children co-opted sensory deprivation to provide a scientific basis for their cutting-edge pedagogic methods.

Head Start Evaluation

While the stated goals of the Head Start program were to prevent cultural deprivation and to promote school readiness, how to evaluate the program's results was from the outset a subject of fierce controversy and debate.[124] Most of the early studies on the effects of Project Head Start examined whether the children's IQs had been raised, a parameter easy to quantify and isolate but not necessarily reflective of the program's goals.[125] Head Start, which had been greeted with much bipartisan support at its inception, was seen as holding promise for a rapid solution for a long-standing problem—the achievement gap between children of different socioeconomic and ethnic backgrounds. While some child development experts openly criticized what they termed "get enrichment quick" schemes, many were won over by the promise of using scientific expertise to make a tangible difference in low-income children's lives.[126]

The program enjoyed federal funding and wide public support, but maintaining them would require proving that the program delivered what it promised. Educational researchers quickly launched evaluation programs funded by federal grants, most often from the OEO and the NIMH. Furthermore, while early enrichment programs had been seen as cutting-edge educational methods in the early and mid-1960s, by later in the decade, the competing theory of "racial isolation" had gained popularity. This theory relied heavily on two major documents. The first, published in 1966, was the *Equality of Educational Opportunity Report.* The 1964 Civil Rights Act had mandated a large-scale comparative evaluation of the public educational facilities available for children from different backgrounds. Johns Hopkins sociologist James Coleman directed the study, and the document it produced is commonly referred to as the Coleman Report. It suggested that inequality between de facto segregated schools was of lesser magnitude than previously estimated, a claim criticized by many African American educators. Furthermore, the Coleman Report suggested that African American children performed better when learning with a white majority, a claim that gained popularity because it suggested that desegregation in itself had educational value. The second document was *Racial Isolation in the Public Schools*, a 1967 U.S. Commission on Civil Rights study of de facto segregation practices.[127] Both reports showed that African American children in desegregated schools achieved higher scholastic outcomes. The "racial isolation" of children in segregated classes was blamed for their low scholastic performance, and some educators argued that desegregation alone was the way to fix the achievement gap. Accordingly, educators and politicians argued that simply placing African American children in white-majority classes could rectify educational inequality.[128]

This seemingly simple solution, which transformed the political question of the implementation of widespread desegregation into an educational question, had much appeal. Desegregation, previously held to be a political and social necessity, was now found to be an effective educational intervention. Furthermore, if desegregated schools improved black scholastic achievement, costly early intervention programs were redundant.[129] Prominent African American leaders, including Kenneth Clark, supported this renewed emphasis on desegregation. In fact, Clark had previously criticized compensatory education as a "cop-out" by perpetuating de facto segregated programs for early enrichment.[130]

The early 1960s enthusiasm for early childhood enrichment was soon eroded by theories of racial isolation and the move toward active desegregation, which received support from liberal politicians, educators, and African American activists. In this context, the evaluation of Head Start was a highly contested field, with not only federal funding and scientific prestige at stake but also the entire theory of compensatory education as a means to close the racial and socioeconomic gaps in scholastic achievement. If compensatory education was proven ineffective, as Arthur Jensen later argued, the accepted environmental theory explaining this gap would be called into question, undercutting the work of antiracist educators and psychologists. Although early evaluation studies attempted to analyze gains in IQ, no robust evidence of such gains was found, and the focus soon shifted to more intangible benefits, such as concepts of school readiness and psychological traits.

Politicians who strongly supported Head Start but had no background in early childhood education hoped that a well-timed intervention could prevent the ravages of poverty and make up for the deficiencies the children had encountered in their early years of life. Edward Zigler has defined this approach as an "inoculation model,"— based on the belief that a measured intervention could produce irreversible changes in a child's development. Zigler has forcefully argued against this idea, writing that it is impossible to "inoculate children in one year against the ravages of a life of deprivation."[131] Zigler's claim has been cited extensively by researchers wanting to emphasize that a single intervention was inadequate and that long-term interventions and structural changes were needed.[132]

In the 1960s, however, immunization became a well-accepted model of a successful public health intervention, and health officials held great hopes in the eradication of certain illnesses through large-scale vaccination projects. The War on Poverty and the eradication campaigns of the 1960s, such as one to "wipe out" measles, shared the belief that both poverty and illness could be effectively targeted through massive intervention.[133] Furthermore, Head Start centers provided childhood vaccinations to children who might not have otherwise had access to primary medical care.[134] Yet I have found no evidence to support Zigler's argument that 1960s child development experts and politicians relied on the inoculation metaphor to support their view of how Head Start protected children against the detrimental effects of poverty. In fact, the only contemporary reference I found to the inoculation model was when it was used as a straw man.[135] Although, as Zigler has argued, many politicians shared the rather unrealistic hope that the short intervention would have significant long-lasting effects, this optimism appears to have been based on a belief in the program's ability to protect children from the perils of deprivation rather than immunizing them against the effects of poverty.

In fact, some researchers pitted the immunization model against the idea of nutritional deprivation. Child psychiatrist Leon Eisenberg and psychologist C. Keith Conners, both at Johns Hopkins, received grants from the OEO and the Grant Foundation of the City of New York to evaluate the effectiveness of a Baltimore Head Start program. Administering tests of cognitive development to children before and after participation in the program and to a control group, Eisenberg and Conners reported significant gains. Yet in questioning the persistence of these gains, the authors noted that one would not "anticipate that a good diet at age 5 would protect a child against malnutrition at age 6"; the mind would require "alimentation" at every stage of development.[136] Eisenberg and Conners preferred the nutritional metaphor over the immunization analogy as a means of advocating on behalf of enrichment programs that would continue throughout elementary school.

Many other evaluations relied on images of deprivation. For example, social worker Hilliard E. Chesteen Jr. evaluated a summer Head Start program in Baton Rouge, Louisiana. Chesteen's study, which was funded by the OEO, devoted more than seventy pages to attempting to define and describe the culturally deprived child. Chesteen uncritically cited both sensory deprivation studies and descriptions of maternal functioning in matrifocal families as well as research on nutritional deprivation.[137] He similarly relied on deprivation theory to offer positive interpretations of the different findings his research unveiled. When Chesteen's study found that the children scored highest in the verbal field in tests administered before the intervention and showed the smallest improvement following intervention, he interpreted these results as evidence that "verbal stimulation" in the children's home environment was higher than other forms of stimulation there. The verbal enrichment the children received was less effective because they were less deprived in this area.[138] His findings, Chesteen argued, highlighted "the lack of stimulation in the living experience of the culturally deprived child," which was the cause of clear educational deficiencies. Preschool intervention could be beneficial in reversing these deficiencies and would be in the best interest of both the deprived children and their future schoolteachers, since Head Start would lead to better-prepared children in elementary school classrooms.[139]

The OEO commissioned the Ohio-based Westinghouse Learning Corporation to prepare a comprehensive evaluation of Head Start's first four years. The report, published in 1969, was deeply polarizing in professional and political circles and has been criticized as being flawed in both design and methodology. The report found no gains in "cognitive and affective development" among children who participated in the summer program and only modest cognitive gains among children who had completed a full-year program.[140] Many Nixon administration officials embraced this critical report. Daniel Patrick Moynihan saw the report as offering an opportunity to reevaluate a program that although popular, might not be "working so well after all," while a high-ranking OEO evaluator questioned whether "we are putting our money in the right place."[141] Child development experts worried that the report would lead to the end of Project Head Start or a significant cut in its funding and immediately criticized the Nixon administration for overplaying the report's negative findings.[142] Stanford University researcher William G. Madow, who participated in the early stages of the report, wrote to request that his name be removed "since I would not want anyone to think I had any responsibility for the design, and the analyses and conclusions based on them seem to me to be incorrect." Child development experts wrote anguished letters to newspaper editors and politicians to protest the report's findings.[143] Although Head Start survived this negative evaluation, the report had a long-lasting effect on public opinion regarding the program's value as well as the wisdom of large-scale interventions targeting minority and low-income children.[144]

Head Start's supporters argued that the report's findings were based on questionable statistical analyses and used irrelevant criteria to define effectiveness. As child development experts strove to dispel the doubts raised by the report, a nutritional model was often invoked. Developmental psychologist Sheldon White wrote that "if the Headstart child is really intellectually undernourished in his environment, then he lives in this environment 24 hours a day for six years. . . . [I]t is unreasonable to expect [the program] to be totally, or perhaps even meaningfully compensatory."[145] Others faulted the report for failing to take into account the important role of the program's nutritional component.[146] Perceptions of deprivation not only served as the theoretical basis for the intervention but also provided a framework through which to interpret its results and to rebut studies claiming to show minimal long-term benefits from the intervention.

Child development experts ultimately helped reformulate Project Head Start's goals, shifting the focus away from questions of IQ to more holistic measures of "social competence" and "school readiness." These parameters were harder to isolate and quantify but better reflected the program's benefits.[147] By the mid-1970s, the program also distanced itself from terms such as "cultural deprivation," which by that time had become controversial.[148] Instead, Head Start relied solely on descriptions of socioeconomic disadvantage, recasting the program as a means to prepare children for school. Head Start gradually shifted its focus from developing intelligence to preparing children for school. This transition was completed with the 1998 reauthorization of Head Start, which legally defined "school readiness" as the program's goal and primary outcome measure. This goal led to new guidelines for receiving funding: For example, 50 percent of the educational staff would have an least an associate's degree, and math- and reading-readiness material had to be included in the curriculum. In addition, for-profit organizations were for the first time permitted to compete for Head Start funds.[149] The shift from promoting intellectual development and compensating for perceived deprivations to preparing young children for school was reflected in the transition from programs designed to provide an educational environment comparable to a stimulating middle-class home to an attempt to provide toddlers with an academic, school-like environment.

Conclusion

Perceptions of deprivation were closely tied to those of race. Gray and Klaus's Early Training Program and Martin Deutsch's IDS served only African American children; the MFY targeted Latino and African American families. Project Head Start targeted children from low-income families, a group that included disproportionate numbers of African Americans. Although Head Start has always served more white American children than African Americans, the percentage of blacks enrolled has always been disproportionately high, as has the percentage of African American paraprofessionals employed by Head Start, many of them parents of participating children.[150]

In the South, Head Start was identified with African Americans, and the most famous of the southern programs was the Child Development Group of Mississippi (CDGM). The state of Mississippi refused to apply for Head Start funding because federal money would have mandated the establishment of desegregated facilities. In response, public, private, and church-affiliated organizations united to create the CDGM and apply for Head Start funding. In 1965, they received $1.5 million, the second-largest grant awarded that year. The CDGM was unique in its wholehearted adoption of the model of maximum feasible participation, relying on the African American community it served for both planning and implementation. This program aroused the wrath of its white supremacist opponents, who went to great lengths to jeopardize the program's federal funding with allegations of fiscal misconduct. In addition, crosses were burned and shots were fired at the Mississippi Head Start center, and local law enforcement agents issued nuisance traffic tickets and harassed local participants and activists. The Mississippi experience certainly contributed to white families' reluctance to send their children to Head Start centers and helped shape Project Head Start's identification with low-income children of color.[151]

All of these early intervention programs shared the assumption that the children they targeted were deprived of adequate maternal care and necessary sensory stimulation and were suffering from inadequate diets. Removing young children from their unstimulating homes, placing them in an environment rich in perceptual stimulation under the care of teachers who provided adequate care for intellectual development, and feeding them nutritious food were integral parts of these different interventions.

Politics went hand in hand with child development theory, as deprivation theory was used to justify federally funded intervention, interpret its results, and deflect unfavorable findings. In contrast, HARYOU, an African American community action program, eschewed deprivation theory in favor of explanations in line with the group's own political agenda, faulting biased teachers and inadequate schools for providing insufficient educational opportunities. Ironically, the MFY's educational leaders, who promoted a controversial program designed to empower and mobilize low-income and minority communities, displayed perhaps the lowest opinion of low-income mothers and the stimulation they provided their children.

While "culturally deprived" had been recognized as a euphemism for describing low-income African Americans since the early 1960s, the term also took part in public discourse on color blindness. In describing the detrimental effects of growing up in poverty and the long-lasting effects of deprivation, researchers and politicians shifted the focus away from questions of race. Although time and again interventions using federal funds targeted African American children, any discussion of race was superseded by a focus on socioeconomic status. If the unique problems of African American children were mentioned, it was usually in passing, and such problems were depicted as an additional disadvantage beyond that of living in poverty. Other observers simply noted the focus on African American children as a decision made out of convenience as a consequence of location and availability. Yet ignoring race did not make it disappear. Kenneth Clark argued in 1967 that these enrichment programs were not a form of "compensatory" education but simply demonstrated that with efficient teaching, African American children could learn as rapidly their white counterparts. These programs, he argued, should be understood as the contemporary version of "separate but equal education." Rather than providing adequate education for all children regardless of race, enrichment programs provided a separate system to provide what should be universally available. These programs, he argued, "obscure the basic fact that underprivileged children are being systematically shortchanged in their regular segregated and inferior schools."[152]

Shifting the focus onto the discrete components of stimulation that African American children were seen as lacking and providing these elements through federally funded interventions enabled educators and politicians to circumvent a serious discussion of the implications of growing up black and poor in the United States. Deprivation was seen as a barrier to success that could be mitigated by appropriate educational intervention, thus avoiding an analysis of the social factors that led to the high poverty rates in African American communities. Well-intentioned and based on state-of-the-art child development theory, these early intervention programs certainly had many benefits for the children and the greater community they served. Showing how these intervention programs were based on a framework of nutritional, maternal, and sensory deprivation does not necessarily question their historical importance and value. In fact, as education historian Diane Ravitch has argued, "compensatory education program" was a misnomer: these programs simply provided a good early childhood education.[153] Yet this analysis provides insight on the preconceptions of liberal politicians and liberal-minded child development experts, who colluded to create a coherent theory of cultural deprivation and its perceived remedy through enrichment. This approach demonstrates the pitfalls of using science to avoid addressing pressing social and economic problems.

CHAPTER FOUR

Deprivation and Intellectual Disability
From "Mild Mental Retardation" to Resegregation

IN THE LATE 1950S AND 1960S, child mental health experts created a new category of disability: "mild mental retardation" caused by deprivation.[1] Profoundly influencing public policy, this diagnosis was as a highly political category and had far-reaching practical implications.[2] The diagnosis of "mild mental retardation" was often the first step in placing children in separate tracks or special education classes in their schools. Since the late 1960s, the category of mild intellectual disability has been the subject of much controversy, as it has been disproportionately used to diagnose racial and ethnic minorities as well as children from low-income homes. This diagnostic disparity remains evident today.

As disability scholars have noted, "special education" classes serving the black poor provide inadequate educational services and have low exit rates, meaning that few children rejoin the mainstream educational system. In contrast, less stigmatizing categories such as "learning disabled" function as a category of "privilege for the privileged," guaranteeing mainly white students access to services and accommodations such as extra time in testing situations or one-on-one tutoring.[3] Disability scholar Christine Sleeter has argued that learning disabilities, as opposed to the categories of "mental retardation" and "cultural deprivation," emerged in the 1960s as a privileged category to describe white middle-class children falling behind in an increasingly demanding school system while differentiating them from low-income African American children. In contrast, diagnoses of intellectual disability have been disproportionately employed for more than five decades to describe children of color. These diagnoses have consistently resulted in decreased access to general education and lower rates of transition to mainstream classes.

This disturbing overrepresentation of low-income and minority children in special education can be traced back to the early 1960s.[4] During this period of early desegregation, African American children with diverse educational backgrounds joined schools that had been racially and socioeconomically homogenous. White educators viewed the academic performance of many of these children—below that of many of their white peers—as a marker for intellectual disability. Yet this diagnosis would not have been possible had deprivation not been established as an etiological factor for intellectual disability.

This chapter examines how deprivation theory provided the scientific basis for the wide diagnosis of "mild mental retardation" among low-income African American children. While ostensibly designed to identify children with special needs and tailor appropriate intervention, the resultant over-diagnosis led to de facto segregated classes grouped accordingly to perceived ability and the resulting denial of appropriate educational opportunities. Deprivation theory facilitated this unfortunate outcome.

Psychiatrists and psychologists revised the classifications of intellectual disability to reflect current theories of deprivation. Concepts of maternal and sensory deprivation rather than the ill-defined "cultural deprivation" determined how physicians, psychologist, and educators viewed intellectual disability. The discourse on deprivation as a causal factor in intellectual disability was reflected in the Kennedy administration's attempts to implement a national plan for combating intellectual disability. I evaluate three different intervention programs developed on the basis of the deprivation hypothesis, one earlier, in which race was not addressed, and two from the mid- to late 1960s that exclusively targeted African American children. Finally, I examine how theories of cultural deprivation and "mild mental retardation" facilitated the overrepresentation of African Americans in special education classes and evaluate later critiques of the use of these diagnoses as means to resegregate recently desegregated schools into racially homogenous classes.

Classifications of Intellectual Disability

Deprivation made its first appearance as diagnostic category in intellectual disability in the 1959 manual of the American Association on Mental Deficiency (AAMD) and subsequently appeared in the revisions of the *International Classification of Disease*, 8th edition (*ICD 8*) (1967), and in the *Diagnostic and Statistical Manual of Mental Diseases*, 2nd edition (*DSM II*) (1968). Significantly, deprivation had not appeared in any form in earlier diagnoses of intellectual disability or in the earlier versions of the *ICD* and the *DSM*. Within a decade, deprivation appeared as an etiological factor in all three major classifications of intellectual disability, demonstrating the profound impact deprivation theory had on the mental health profession.

In 1959, the AAMD, the leading professional organization for the study of intellectual disability, published its first *Manual on Terminology and Classification*, formulated by Richard F. Heber, a child psychologist and researcher in the field of intellectual disability. The manual served as the foremost diagnostic classification of intellectual disability at the time and was the first to include deprivation as an etiological factor, providing the basis for the later inclusion of deprivation by both the *ICD 8* and the *DSM II*.[5] Prior to publication of the *AAMD Manual*, researchers and clinicians had relied on different and nonstandardized forms of diagnosis and classification, mostly based on presumed etiology or on level of functioning.[6]

The definition of "mental retardation" presented in the *AAMD Manual* relied on performance at a level lower than one standard deviation below the mean in tests designed to measure intelligence, a cutoff considered quite inclusive, even at the time. The manual was revised in 1961 to include the criterion of "adaptive behavior." Although not clearly defined in Heber's text, this term was taken mainly to refer to individuals' ability to conduct themselves independently in the world, closely tied to concepts of intellectual and emotional maturity. This revision slightly restricted the definition, which could no longer rely solely on the results of intelligence testing.[7] This definition remained in use until the publication of the 1973 revision of the *Manual on Terminology and Classification in Mental Retardation*, which required a measured IQ of more than two standard deviations below the mean, thus substantially decreasing the number of individuals classified as "mentally retarded."[8]

In Heber's introduction to the *AAMD Manual*, he addressed the controversy over the role of nonorganic "psychogenic and psychosocial factors" in causing intellectual disability. As a form of compromise, he proposed a group of diagnoses under the heading "mental retardation due to uncertain (or presumed psychologic) cause with the functional reaction alone manifest."[9] This group of "uncertain" causes that could lead to intellectual disability included two diagnoses based on deprivation, "cultural-familial mental retardation" and "psychogenic mental retardation associated with environmental deprivation." The first category required a similarly afflicted family member (parent or sibling) and was defined as often being accompanied by "parental inadequacy" leading to some degree of "cultural deprivation." Thus, cultural deprivation was held to be a cause of intellectual disability and was caused at least in part by "parental inadequacy." Again, theories of cultural deprivation relied on models of better-established forms of deprivation such as maternal deprivation.

In the second category, "psychogenic mental retardation associated with environmental deprivation," Heber referred both to deprivation of learning experiences seen to be "essential for adequate functioning in our culture" and to deprivation of stimulation, including cases of "severe sensory impairments such as blindness and deafness, or rarely, as the result of severe environmental restrictions or highly atypical cultural experience."[10] Different forms of deprivation, ranging from a lack of educational opportunities to a form of "sensory deprivation" caused by organic disability, were grouped together as potential causes of intellectual disability.[11]

In the 1960s, revisions of both the *ICD* and the *DSM* included the category of mental retardation caused by deprivation.[12] As noted by psychiatrists Robert Spitzer and Paul Wilson, who participated in the *DSM*'s revision, the new category of mental retardation "with psychosocial (environmental) deprivation" in the *DSM II* reflected new ways of thinking about the causes of mental retardation.[13] Under the category of "mental retardation with psychosocial (environmental) deprivation" were two subheadings, identical to the AAMD 1959 classification: "cultural familial mental retardation" and "psychogenic mental retardation associated with environmental deprivation."[14] Environmental deprivation was given a very broad interpretation, as the *DSM* text noted that deprivation resulting from "severe sensory impairment" may occur even in an environment that seems rich in stimulation or can result from environmental constrictions or "atypical cultural milieus."[15] "Mental retardation" secondary to deprivation could be diagnosed in a wide variety of situations. Wilson and Spitzer gave the example of a patient with "chronic undifferentiated schizophrenia who has mild mental retardation attributable to a pathological situation." Under the diagnostic framework of the *DSM II*, this patient would receive two diagnoses, one of schizophrenia, "chronic undifferentiated type," and the other of "mild mental retardation with psychosocial (environmental) deprivation."[16]

Thus, the rise of deprivation theory led to the creation of a new diagnostic category: intellectual disability caused by deprivation. Firmly established within mainstream mental health discourse, deprivation-based views of intellectual disability profoundly influenced public policy.

Intellectual Disability and Public Policy

The early 1960s heralded an era of unprecedented public and governmental interest in the question of intellectual disability. Previously seen as an unattractive field for research or funding, with each state adopting different practices for the custodial care of children with special needs, the diagnosis and treatment of children with intellectual disabilities came to the forefront during this decade.[17] A number of factors contributed to this change; in particular, activist groups of parents of children with disabilities demanded better services for their children. In the early 1950s, parents began to share their experiences of caring for children with special needs, leading to the emergence of a distinct confessional genre of popular books and articles. Well-educated, middle-class white parents depicted their children as "angels" or as "children who never grow up" and bemoaned the lack of adequate facilities to assist in their care. Parents first organized to create local groups, which ultimately came together in 1950 to establish the National Association for Retarded Children, one of the most powerful lobbying groups of the time.[18] Furthermore, the Cold War led to a renewed interest in how to better educate children and improve their intellectual abilities, with America's strength measured by its population's perceived intellectual and scientific abilities.[19] Scholastic success was seen to be part and parcel of U.S. international and military interests, a theme reflected in many popular journals at the time. A 1961 *Saturday Evening Post* article warned that what Soviet and American students learn in school "may do much to determine whether the free world will check and defeat Communism, or whether Communism will check and defeat the free world."[20] This emphasis on scholastic ability, which was profoundly shaped by the Cold War and the high value placed on science, led experts to examine why certain children were falling behind. Barriers to academic achievement were seen as a pressing public concern.

The Kennedy family's long-standing interest in the care of children with intellectual disabilities was undoubtedly influenced by their personal experience with President John F. Kennedy's sister, Rosemary Kennedy, who had been diagnosed with such a disability. The members of the Kennedy family were willing to share their experiences with the public, thus introducing the challenge of dealing with a child with intellectual disabilities into American households.[21] The Kennedys' activism in the field of intellectual disability significantly contributed to the public discourse on the topic and buoyed a powerful lobby for the cause.[22] The Joseph P. Kennedy Jr. Foundation, es-

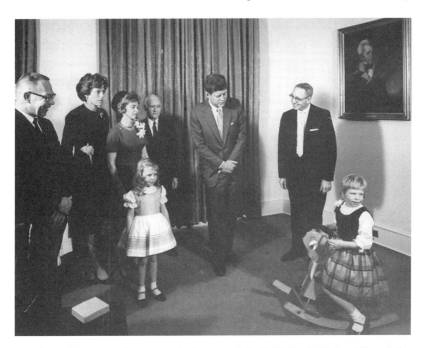

President John F. Kennedy meets with Kammy and Sheila McGrath, National Retarded Children's Week poster children for 1961. Photo by Abbie Rowe. Courtesy of White House Photographs, John F. Kennedy Presidential Library and Museum, Boston.

tablished in 1946, developed an influential program in intellectual disability research, enlisting key figures nationwide.[23] Eunice Kennedy Shriver, another of President Kennedy's sisters, was one of the driving forces behind efforts to improve the care available for individuals with intellectual disabilities. In 1961, the president published a call for action, articulating the need for a nationwide program to address "mental retardation" and focusing particularly on the need for prevention. In this statement, Kennedy outlined the accepted view of intellectual disability, which he argued was not a disease but rather a symptom of various conditions, including "mongolism, birth injury or infection, or even inadequate stimulation in early childhood."[24] The specific mentioning of inadequate stimulation (tantamount to deprivation) demonstrates the wide dissemination and acceptance of this new etiological factor in the causation of intellectual disability.

Kennedy then established the President's Panel on Mental Retardation, headed by educator and intellectual disability specialist Leonard Mayo. Members of this panel collected and evaluated data on the treatment and prevention of intellectual disability in the United States and abroad. The collection and interpretation of information were profoundly shaped by the political climate. In 1962, six members of the panel spent three weeks in the Soviet Union observing research and treatment facilities for the intellectually disabled. Samuel Kirk, a University of Illinois researcher on intellectual disability, and his protégé, Lloyd Dunn, director of special education at Tennessee's Peabody College, highlighted the differences between the Soviet and the American approaches: Soviet scientists viewed all intellectual disability to be physiological, rejecting theories of "cultural causation." Since every Soviet child was believed to be exposed to identical cultural surroundings, Lloyd and Dunn explained, Soviet experts discounted any possibility of environmental influences on intellectual development. Rates of intellectual disability in the Soviet Union were estimated at between a half and one-third of those for the United States. To explain this discrepancy, the authors hypothesized that the "rapid clearing" of "slums" in the Soviet Union and greater equality in the standard of living contributed to a lower rate of disability. Furthermore, the authors suggested that "cultural deprivation may also be reduced for Russian children of lower socioeconomic status by the availability and frequent use made of the Palaces of Culture, museums, ballets, operas, summer camps for children, etc."[25] To further highlight the interrelations of social factors and the prevalence of intellectual disability, the authors cited the findings of a mission to Scandinavian countries similarly sponsored by the panel: There was "half the amount of mental retardation in Denmark and Sweden as in our country," results that the report's authors suggested might stem from "less cultural deprivation, more tax-supported medical services, and a lower rate of prematurity." In this instance, theories of intellectual disability were enlisted to promote a liberal political agenda.

In October 1962, the President's Panel on Mental Retardation submitted its report, *A Proposed Program for National Action to Combat Mental Retardation*. Examining different aspects of the prevention and treatment of mental retardation, the report demonstrated a clear acceptance of the theory of deprivation as an etiological factor in intellectual disability. Furthermore, the report facilely tied together different forms of deprivation, blurring distinctions among them. For example, the introduction argued, "The majority of the mentally retarded are the children of the more disadvantaged classes of our society. . . . A number of experiments with the education of presumably retarded children from slum neighborhoods strongly suggest that a predominant cause of mental retardation may be the lack of learning opportunities or absence of 'intellectual vitamins' under these adverse environmental conditions."[26] This paragraph implied that poverty and life in a "slum" neighborhood caused mental retardation, thus alluding to common theories of cultural deprivation. The concept of "intellectual vitamins" as a commodity reflects perceptions of poverty and its perils and the widespread acceptance of the idea. A 1964 article in the *New York Times* cited a theory of intellectual disability that found that "childhood performance on a level of retardation may take place at least temporarily because of a lack of 'intellectual vitamins.'"[27]

The report argued that many "mentally retarded" individuals had been deprived of the stimulation and learning opportunities necessary for the development of intelligence.[28] The authors examined the epidemiology of cultural deprivation and its financial implications in terms of lost productivity and suggested the establishment of preschool enrichment centers that would instill in "deprived" children the "attitudes and aptitudes" that middle-class children naturally developed, which were seen as pivotal for academic success. In fact, these centers were proposed to "become a part of the public school system" in underprivileged areas so that children from low-income homes could effectively start "school" before age three.[29]

In what might seem to be a surprising transition, the next section of the report was devoted to the potentially detrimental effects of maternal deprivation and separation. First citing findings regarding the detrimental effects of institutionalization, the report commended the positive changes that had been made to avoid maternal deprivation—foster care placement or the provision of more individual attention in cases of institutional care.[30] Apart from these extreme situations, the authors also cited more mundane examples of potentially damaging maternal separation, including what they termed the "unavailable mother"—a mother who did not provide her child with what was seen to be necessary care for reasons that could include maternal employment or "emotional unavailability."[31]

Early child care for lower-class children, including the suggestion to begin nursery school education at the age of three years, was not depicted as a cause of maternal deprivation but rather as an intervention designed to prevent deprivation. This class-based distinction was common at the time; early enrichment programs for children from low-income families were not cited as a cause of maternal deprivation. Thus, the report recommended different interventions by local and state health and welfare agencies that could contribute to the "attack upon those particular adverse characteristics of the life of the culturally deprived" that were seen as leading to decreased scholastic and employment success. These interventions included the establishment of day care centers for "young children of working mothers and otherwise 'unavailable' mothers" as well as the provision of "homemakers and home economists to mothers who require help in family and child care." Methods by which to prevent cultural deprivation, an accepted etiological factor in intellectual disability, were based on class-stratified perceptions of normative mothering.

This report provided the scientific basis for federal action. In February 1963, President Kennedy addressed Congress, presenting his vision for tackling the "twin problems" of mental illness and mental retardation. He delineated three main objectives—preventing mental illness and mental retardation, increasing the resources of knowledge and trained professionals in the field, and improving the available programs and facilities. Directly addressing questions of race and class, the president made the somewhat contradictory statement that "mental retardation strikes children without regard for class, creed or economic level" but it hit the underprivileged and poor harder and more often.[32] Referring to the "self-perpetuating intellectual blight" of children from low-income areas who lacked the "stimulus" necessary for intellectual development, Kennedy described his vision for providing educational opportunities in "slum and distressed areas." These interventions would "help prevent mental retardation among the children in such culturally deprived areas." The discourse of deprivation as an etiological cause for intellectual disability clearly had attained acceptability up to the highest policymaking level.

Two major pieces of legislation transformed this speech into action. The Maternal and Child Health and Mental Retardation Planning Amendment to the Social Security Act, signed in October 1963, provided funding for states to update their programs for individuals with intellectual disabilities as well as increasing funding for prevention by providing maternal and early infant care. The Community Mental Health Act, signed later the same month, provided federal funding for community-based mental health facilities. Both proposals were accepted enthusiastically by physicians, including psychiatrists, pediatricians, obstetricians, and public health specialists.[33] These acts ultimately hastened the controversial process known as "deinstitutionalization," in which the site of mental care was transformed from long-term residential institutions to care in the community itself.[34]

Deprivation and Intellectual Disability

The rise of deprivation as a distinct etiological factor in intellectual disability reflected its growing acceptance both in medical and social policy discourse. Throughout the 1960s, physicians and researchers began examining the etiology, prevention, and treatment of intellectual disability through a focus on deprivation and deficiencies. Most publications examining "mild mental retardation" also included an analysis of these children's socioeconomic class. Significantly, few articles addressed the question of race, although a disproportionate number of the children diagnosed as suffering from "mild mental retardation" were African American. Rather, during the civil rights era, researchers and politicians propounded a "color-blind" approach that examined what forms of deprivation caused "mental retardation" and how they could be prevented. Numerous articles examined what children from poor families lacked and how these gaps determined their mental capacities. Researchers increasingly chose to refer to deprivations in the plural, reflecting a broad perception of what might be lacking.

By the early 1950s, the Group for the Advancement of Psychiatry (GAP), founded in 1946, had become an influential advisory organization dedicated to shaping psychiatric thinking and public policy by publishing reports and position statements on key topics concerning the intersection of mental health and society. In a 1959 report, *Basic Considerations in Mental Retardation*, GAP declared that "complex physical and psychological deprivations" were central in the etiology of "mild mental retardation." The report enumerated the hazards of "poor nutrition, unhygienic environment, general neglect, inadequate mothering and lack of intellectual stimulation," presenting an all-embracing depiction of deprivation as not only an important etiological factor but also the essence of disadvantaged children's home lives.[35]

This view persisted throughout the 1960s, as psychiatrists and child development experts highlighted the dangers of low-income children's deficient home environments. Some observers quite clearly sought to identify missing elements. One experimental psychologist wrote to psychologist Joseph McVicker Hunt explaining his interest in examining how the "normal" child learns, since "if we know what the normal child has 'got' we might better be able to find ou[t] what the retarded child 'hasn't got.'"[36]

Like Kennedy, psychiatrists saw poverty as an important factor in intellectual disability. Psychiatrist Joseph Wortis, a longtime scholar of intellectual disability, wrote that "the poor tend to be intellectually undernourished. . . . [T]he conventional family unit is usually not known; the father is often non-existent or absent, the mother is out working or the child lives with a grandmother." Again relying on the nutritional metaphor, Wortis paralleled intellectual deficiency with a deficiency in family structure.[37] Similarly, special education expert Burton Blatt's concept of deprivation encompassed the child's physical environment: "In the homes of disadvantaged families there is a scarcity of furniture and appliances of all types. . . . The families are often nonverbal, i.e., there is little meaningful language used, and the language that is used is frequently unacceptable in nondeprived settings, such as the school. In general, the home and the contiguous neighborhood provide children with a limited range of stimuli and encouragement for exploration and discovery."[38] The different aspects of home life Blatt found wanting were tied to the etiology of mental retardation, implying that the entire home life of these children was deficient. Thus, a lack of furniture was placed on the same scale as a lack of stimulation. This is typical of publications of the time, in which the home environment of the perceived "deprived" children of low socioeconomic status was often described in bleak and stereotypical terms.

In the preface to a 1969 book bearing the unambiguous title *Poverty and Mental Retardation: A Causal Relationship*, Senator Edward M. Kennedy, brother of the late president, described impoverished children as lacking medication, "the right food," and "a house that protects its inhabitants from cold weather and from mosquitoes and flies and rats."[39] Conceptualizing possible exposure to cold weather and rodents as a form of lack or deprivation rather than a surplus of unwanted components required a considerable commitment to the theory of deprivation. The singular focus on deficiencies and deprivation as etiological factors in intellectual disability shaped how politicians and mental health experts alike viewed low-income children's home lives.

This medicalized, deprivation-based interpretation of low scholastic achievement was reflected in the professional discourse of educators. Herbert Goldstein, an educator at the University of Illinois's Institute for Research on Exceptional Children, edited a short pamphlet on the "educable mentally retarded" elementary school child that was published as part of a series titled "What Research Says to the Teacher." These brief nontechnical pamphlets published by the American Educational Research Association were designed to summarize the state of current relevant research in a manner easily digestible by classroom teachers. In response to the question "What are retarded children like?," Goldstein described what he saw as their obvious "physical and cultural undernourishment": Many were "prone to illness and lacking in physical stamina." "Their language," he continued, "is often impoverished," while a "lack of motivation in schoolwork" resulted from the "family's apathy or lack of understanding of the purposes of education."[40] Medical research on the detrimental effects of different forms of deprivation was seen as directly relevant to classroom educators. Furthermore, a clear continuity existed between perceived physical and social deficits. The entire perception of the low-income families was based on what was seen to be lacking—adequate nutrition, motivation, and comprehension of middle-class values.

While the first GAP report devoted to the question of intellectual disability referred to the multitude of deprivations that afflicted these children, another report, published eight years later, specifically focused on class differences. *Mild Mental Retardation: A Growing Challenge to the Physician* differentiated between two groups of affected children, children growing up in what were portrayed as typical middle-class families and children from low-income homes, whose depiction was almost a caricature. The groups, however, are identified only as A and B, a decision the authors explained as designed to "avoid labels," making no mention of the children's race or ethnicity.[41] Still, to resolve any ambiguity regarding the socioeconomic strata of the groups, the authors emphasized that the "parents of the children in Group A are often uncomfortable in our predominantly middle-class society." The members of Group B lived mainly in the suburbs, while Group A children lived in the inner cities.[42] This distinction corresponded with race: Most inner cities were almost entirely African American, while suburbs were unmistakably white.[43] Group A children's lives were characterized by "dullness, colorlessness and drabness," leading to apathy. In contrast, the parents of the Group B children were more "concerned about their [children], noting [their] deficiencies earlier and taking an active role in seeking medical assistance." Group A mothers were described as depriving, and their children were said to suffer from "insufficient or discontinuous mothering with physical neglect," which contributed to the development of mild intellectual disability.[44] In contrast, Group B parents "may overstimulate the child and develop emotional problems over his failure to respond."[45] Thus, the report suggested two separate etiologies for the same clinical picture of "mild mental retardation." Low-income African American children were deprived and neglected; middle-class suburban children were overstimulated and pushed beyond their abilities. This distinction was maintained throughout the entire report.

Many mental health experts held deprivation to be one of the most important topics in the field of intellectual disability. When invited to serve as chair of the Kansas Governor's Committee on Mental Retardation, Menninger Clinic psychologist Lois Barclay Murphy, a consultant to Head Start, accepted only on the condition that the committee be free to debate a wide range of factors implicated in intellectual disability, including "cultural deprivation."[46] Throughout the committee's meetings, Murphy highlighted the interconnections between a lack of maternal care and malnutrition in the etiology of intellectual disability, showing pictures of children in Nigerian orphanages suffering from marasmus, a severe form of protein deficiency. At the time, the term "marasmus" was also used to describe the condition of institutionalized children who suffered from a failure to thrive for a variety of reasons, including maternal deprivation.[47] Elsewhere Murphy enumerated the different forms of deprivation that could lead to "mental deficiency": a lack of sensory stimulation, nutritional deficiencies, and maternal deprivation, including insufficient skin contact with the mother's body.[48] Not surprisingly, the task force she chaired suggested an early education program designed to provide sensory stimulation, screen for sensory deficiencies, and provide nutritious food as well as individualized attention in blocks of ten to fifteen minutes to simulate the care that should have been provided by an attentive mother. All of these measures were designed to compensate for the deprivations seen to lead to intellectual disability.[49]

While some researchers focused on a multitude of forms of deprivation as salient in the etiology of intellectual deprivation, others implicated a single form. Many researchers touted maternal deprivation, long believed to hinder intellectual development, as a major cause of mental retardation. While most maternal deprivation theorists viewed the nursery school teacher as a mother-substitute who could provide much-needed individualized attention and education, others, such as psychoanalyst René Spitz, went so far as to suggest that the adoption of intellectually disabled children "by someone with maternal feelings will do wonders."[50] Both John Bowlby and Mary Ainsworth highlighted the importance of studies on maternal deprivation in the development of the field of intellectual disability and the therapeutic aspects of providing adequate maternal care via trained caregivers.[51]

Others viewed sensory deprivation as the sole cause of mild mental retardation.[52] George Tarjan, a University of California at Los Angeles psychiatrist and influential researcher in the field of intellectual disability, had served as a consultant to the Joseph P. Kennedy Jr. Foundation, was a founding member of the President's Committee on Mental Retardation, and later served as president of the American Psychiatric Association. At a 1968 symposium on "Psychodynamic Implications of the Studies in Sensory Deprivation," held at the Eastern Pennsylvania Psychiatric Institute, Tarjan linked three childhood syndromes to sensory deprivation: sociocultural retardation, the symptom complex of early childhood psychosis, and the sequelae of prematurity.[53] Sensory deprivation permeated psychiatric discourse, becoming an influential framework by which to interpret a number of conditions that today would commonly be considered unrelated.

Children with "sociocultural" intellectual disability, Tarjan argued, were "often unplanned, unwanted, or illegitimate and are reared in environments with absent fathers and physically or emotionally unavailable mothers. They are left unattended for long periods and are not exposed to the tactile and kinesthetic stimulations customary for middle-class children. There are sounds, sights and odors in their surroundings, but these sensory stimuli are not as organized or coordinated as those in the average environment. For instance, the sounds are mostly noise and the children usually hear only brief words of negative connotations."[54] Tarjan's negative view of low-income homes and their role in causing intellectual disability is striking: The home environment itself and the supposed inadequacy of the parents were seen as pathogenic. Although specifically referring to sensory deprivation as the significant factor in this form of "sociocultural retardation," Tarjan highlighted the dangers of the absent father and inadequate mother, demonstrating the inseparability of sensory and maternal deprivation. Even when researchers made a point of isolating one form of deprivation, the other nearly always appeared in some form.

That same year, Tarjan also participated in an international conference jointly organized by Peabody College and the National Institute of Mental Health (NIMH) on "Social-Cultural Aspects of Mental Retardation." At this conference, which emphasized environmental factors in intellectual disability, Tarjan stated that "the theory currently most generally accepted by American scientists bases the etiology of sociocultural retardation on [a] model of stimulus deprivation."[55]

At a time when intellectual disability was receiving much political attention, policymakers turned to experts to seek guidance. Physicians, psychologists, and social scientists lent their scientific authority to governmental committees and federally funded interventions. In 1966, Lyndon Baines Johnson established the President's Committee on Mental Retardation (today the President's Committee for People with Intellectual Disabilities), a federal advisory commission that prioritized prevention and early recognition and consisted of politicians, professional experts, and representatives of the lay public. This committee was designed to provide advice on policy issues and submit an annual report to the president. While the first report referred to the surfeit of cases of mental retardation in low-income areas, the second report, published in 1968, included the term "deprivation" in its title. Intellectual disabilities "afflicting millions of Americans," the report argued, "stem from neglect, deprivation and lack of stimulation during infancy and early childhood." Accordingly, the committee recommended that service agencies, public and private, act immediately to ensure access to health and educational services as a right from birth.[56] The committee members "urge[d] all speed" on the "war on poverty" as part of the attempts to prevent intellectual disability. Tying Johnson's War on Poverty with attempts to prevent intellectual disability, this statement illustrates the interrelations between public health intervention and social policy.[57]

While some researchers used their findings as a rationale to support certain political agendas, others wielded the image of an epidemic of "mental retardation" to influence policymakers. In 1967, Cornell psychologist Urie Bronfenbrenner organized a telegram, funded and signed by thirteen leading child development experts, that was sent to five liberal members of the U.S. Senate who strongly opposed a proposed bill, which was ultimately unsuccessful, that would have used maternal employment as an eligibility criterion for social security benefits. To allow the provision to pass, the signees argued, would "increase problems of mental retardation, school dropouts and delinquency in the coming generation."[58] Maternal employment would lead to maternal deprivation, ultimately resulting in "mental retardation." As intellectual disability was perceived as threatening to American society, these leading child development experts provided politicians with a persuasive scientific argument to strengthen their opposition to a conservative bill that would have decreased eligibility for federal benefits.

Many physicians and child development experts viewed the study of intellectual disability and social policy as inextricably linked. The theme of the AAMD's 1969 annual meeting was "Social Issues and Social Action." Richard Koch, the group's president and a longtime advocate of community care for the disabled, pointedly asked the attendees, "Why should an organization such as ours have had such little social conscience, when day in and day out we deal with the products of that social neglect?" Koch's view of social conscience bore an uncanny resemblance to liberal politics. Calling on the participants to become more politically conscious, he argued that "open housing"—putting an end to racial discrimination in housing—was one of the "single most important aspects of the problem of the ghetto," a step that would contribute to the prevention of intellectual disability. Voicing critiques on topics including abortion policy, race relations, and "the dissipation of funds in Viet Nam," Koch argued that the "AAMD must involve itself in the significant social issues of the day."[59] The association's relevance, according to its president, depended on its engagement with the pressing political questions of the time.

Furthermore, the scientific value of research in the field of intellectual disability was assessed at least in part by its influence on public policy. The degree of influence that research had on public policy was considered a relevant factor by which to judge its importance. Tarjan's colleague, Stanley Wright, sought Julius Richmond's support for Tarjan's unsuccessful nomination for the Albert Lasker Medical Research Award. Wright requested that Richmond address the influence of Tarjan's work on the recommendations of professional agencies and policymakers in general and particularly asked that Richmond consider whether Tarjan's work had contributed to the conceptualization of the Head Start program. Physicians held high regard for the policymaking implications of research in intellectual disability.[60]

Preventing Retardation: Three Intervention Programs

As deprivation became recognized as an etiological factor in intellectual disability, researchers designed preventative interventions to target deprivation. Furthermore, in light of the changes in funding priorities beginning during the Kennedy administration, more funds were available for community-based interventions. These interventions demonstrate how researchers, clinicians, and policymakers viewed the causes of mental retardation and identified potential sites of intervention. This chapter focuses on three programs specifically designed to prevent "mental retardation" by targeting deprivation.

The first project, Children of Deprivation: Changing the Course of Familial Mental Retardation began in 1957 and was based at the University of Iowa. This five-year intervention was financed in part by the U.S. Children's Bureau and the NIMH, and its final report was published in 1967 with a foreword by the head of the Children's Bureau. Led by a pediatrician, Robert Kugel, and a home economist, Mabel Parsons, the project was designed to follow the growth and development of children diagnosed with "familial mental retardation" and to intervene in various areas of their lives and home environment.[61] The children selected for this intervention suffered from "retardation" that "was not due to apparent organic cause, at least one of the parents was also mentally retarded, and the family was from a low socioeconomic group."[62]

These low-income children were sent to an experimental school with a low teacher-student ratio, modern facilities and equipment, and facilities for direct researcher observation. This intervention, although designed for children diagnosed as "mentally retarded," resembled child development experts' contemporary attempts to provide remedial education or educational enrichment for "culturally deprived" children.[63] Yet in light of the proclaimed goal of preventing mental retardation, the home interventions described in the report seem disconnected at best. The home economist developed interventions designed to alter "the unfavorable course of mentally retarded children by enriching their environment." Criticizing the abilities of the children's mothers, the researchers argued that "deficiencies in homemaking techniques were usually quite obvious." The abilities and knowledge of the children's mothers was the subject of four research hypotheses, all held to be relevant to the children's intellectual abilities:

1. The women's housekeeping inadequacies were due more to a lack of knowledge than to lack of interest in their work.
2. These disadvantaged mothers could be motivated to learn good homemaking techniques.
3. These women could be taught some of the necessary skills for improvement of their home environment.
4. The children, their siblings, and the fathers would benefit as the result of the improved abilities of the mothers.[64]

Following these hypotheses, the home economist carried out individual work with the mothers, at least on a weekly basis, to collect information on "budgets, dietary planning, housing, furnishings and clothing," and group meetings and sewing classes were organized.[65] Alas, not all these interventions were equally successful: "Mrs. Frost" was described as a "warm, loving, dirty, common-law wife" who was "unable to profit" from the help offered by the home economist because "she was not interested in being clean."[66] From a current perspective it seems questionable to target the mothers' alleged level of cleanliness in an intervention designed to prevent mental retardation among her children. At the time, however, it reflected the researchers' staunch belief that a wide variety of deficiencies and deprivations caused mental retardation and were a viable and acceptable target for medical and government-funded intervention. This approach also demonstrates the emphasis on the importance of normative middle-class mothering and the tendency to blame mothers for their children's perceived shortcomings. The report concluded by suggesting a "total approach" to alleviating deprivation, questioning whether interventions starting at the age of three might not be too late and instead needed to begin "soon after birth."[67] The program's intrusive attempts to improve low-income children's home lives and their mothers' homemaking abilities were presented as medical interventions relevant to preventing intellectual disability.

In an article in the journal *Children*, Mabel Parsons described her work in the Iowa project. Revealing her view that the entire low-income family was pathological, she described the intervention as targeting "families with mental retardation." She proudly explained that after teaching one mother housekeeping skills in her home, the woman spent six weeks visiting Parsons's house to learn how to care for more "elaborate" homes. Whether the mother was compensated for her cleaning work at Parsons's home remains unclear. When the same woman tearfully confided to Parsons that her husband "was tired of her routine fare and refused to come home for meals," the economist helped her plan menus and order groceries to prepare "the kinds of foods her husband liked."[68] How such activities prevented mental retardation remained unexplained, but Parsons reported overall positive results.

Yet these researchers were not naive. Robert Kugel, who also served on the President's Committee for Mental Retardation, argued in a 1968 lecture for the need to address poverty as a causal factor in "mental retardation." He criticized researchers who "go into the ghetto with our middle-class attitudes and our middle-class experiences and wonder why our good will and professional expertise is met with apathy, indifference or outright hostility." A "growing bitterness" was caused by limited opportunities and structural inequality, he argued, demonstrating his familiarity with the day-to-day challenges low-income families faced. To prevent retardation, Kugel suggested interventions that would provide better health care and social services to low-income areas. Yet in the same lecture, he also referred to the Iowa intervention, lauding Parsons's work: By teaching mothers "about household activities such as sewing, decoration, and cleaning," she was also teaching them "how to help their retarded children."[69] It was possible both to be aware of the structural inequalities and lack of opportunities that characterized the lives of low-income families and to believe in the value of sewing lessons as an intervention designed to address and alleviate "mental retardation."

The second program, now known as the Milwaukee Project, was led by Richard F. Heber, a professor of psychology at the University of Wisconsin, and began in 1966 with generous federal funding. The program targeted infants perceived to be at risk of developing mental retardation because their mothers were both from low-income homes and had received low scores on IQ tests. Initial screenings were performed at well-baby clinics, with complete batteries of IQ tests performed on women identified as meeting the program's criteria. Solely African Americans were targeted because, Howard Garber would later explain, they were the most "predominant and least mobile" in Milwaukee, and the intervention was limited to African American families to "control for cultural and ethnic differences."[70] Apart from this statement, there was no discussion of race in the publications based on the intervention.

Soon after the mothers were discharged from the hospital, the newborns were randomly assigned to either participate in an intensive day care program, which was provided alongside educational interventions aimed at the mothers, or receive no intervention (the control group).[71] Reports of astounding gains in IQ soon appeared in the popular media and in textbooks. However, these reports were not published in any peer-reviewed journal.[72] Despite the fact that Heber's experiments had not undergone the usual review required for scientific acceptance, his findings were widely cited in professional publications, often entirely uncritically.[73] Within a few years, as requests from researchers who contacted Heber about the technical details of the experiment remained unanswered, Heber's findings were questioned.[74] A 1981 scandal involving the massive misappropriation of federal funding for an unrelated project ultimately led to prison terms for Heber and his associates, raising further questions regarding the validity of Heber's work.[75] After his release from prison, Heber did not return to academia, and he died in a 1987 plane crash.[76] This led to much skepticism toward what had been a widely cited experiment.

In the few publications that appeared during the experiment, descriptions of the interventions were conspicuously vague. In a paper delivered in 1970 at a conference of the International Society for Scientific Study of Mental Deficiency, Heber and his colleague, Howard Garber, presented the results of an intervention on forty infants of mothers defined as "mentally retarded," who were compared to controls. Their paper, "Experiment in Prevention of Cultural-Familial Mental Retardation" allegedly tested the "social deprivation hypothesis" of mental retardation.[77] Heber and Garber's research hypothesis demonstrates a mixed approach to deprivation: "The mentally retarded mother residing in the 'slum' creates a social environment for her offspring which is distinctly different from that created by the 'slum-dwelling' mother of normal intelligence." This hypothesis, they admitted, had been reached through "simple observation."[78] Thus, whether a given environment was in fact depriving for the infant depended on the mother's abilities to mold that environment to the child's needs.

Heber's program consisted of two interventions. For the infants, the program was defined as a "customized, precisely structured program of stimulation" that included "essentially every aspect of sensory and language stimulation." The mothers took part in a "rehabilitation" program that involved occupational training alongside training in homemaking and in baby-care techniques. Although the interventions developed in this project ostensibly targeted cultural or social deprivation, they were in fact designed to mitigate the infants' sensory deprivation and to prevent maternal deprivation or maternal inadequacy. In a different description of the program, touted as "one of the most important longitudinal studies ever undertaken," Garber and Heber claimed that the mothers were unaware of the needs of their children. Thus, the researchers argued, the mothers "contribute to the growing number of children so poor in development that they are at high risk for mental retardation"—an explanation that tied together maternal deprivation, cultural deprivation, and intellectual disability.[79]

In 1988, Garber published the first and only comprehensive description of the intervention, providing details about the protocol of stimulation provided for the infants, which was rich and varied. Infants received one-on-one care; each caregiver had only two or three toddlers. One of the caregivers' "major roles" was to provide a "variety of sensory experiences," from different tastes to new smells; other interventions included field trips and music lessons.[80] Reviewing the book, Arthur Jensen recounted an early conversation in which Heber said that this stimulation protocol would make the childhood environments of John Stuart Mill and Sir Francis Galton "very deprived by comparison."[81] Environmental enrichment to prevent sensory deprivation was seen as a key to preventing intellectual disability.

The third intervention was led by child psychiatrist Reginald Lourie and psychologist Dorothy Huntington of the Washington, D.C., Children's Hospital, with psychologist Lois B. Murphy as the senior consultant. Funded by the NIMH between 1965 and 1969, this project was described as an intervention for the "prevention of culturally determined mental retardation."[82] At the time, Lourie headed numerous projects at the Children's Hospital funded by the NIMH and other agencies.[83] Many of these projects had similar names, goals, staff, and intervention components.[84]

Lourie and Huntington's proposal cited the "alarmingly high incidence of mental retardation and personal dysfunction among children growing up in slums" as the impetus for their early intervention program.[85] They suggested a form of day care designed to provide "appropriate stimulation in those areas of development where environmentally induced deficits are often found to be most severe."[86] Again, this intervention was designed only for African American children, a fact explained in a single sentence seven pages into the proposal. The researchers were interested in having "the day care units draw on the population nearby who would receive their medical care at" the Children's Hospital.[87] Deficits accumulated in the first year of life, Lourie and Huntington argued, were largely irreversible after the age of three. If the "stimulation" for the development of personality was "absent or inappropriate," permanent damage, such as "retardation or dysfunction in intelligence, emotional and social functioning," could ensue.[88]

The program also included a component targeting parent-child interaction. This component was based on what the researchers described as a large volume of research that had documented the "meager and repressive infant rearing techniques" in low-income homes. These phenomena were compared to studies on the prolonged institutionalized care of children, and both were said to lead to "retardation of intelligence and social development."[89] In effect, Lourie and Huntington equated what they saw as deficient care provided by low-income parents with the early descriptions of maternal deprivation resulting from prolonged hospitalization. Furthermore, because low-income children were seen as at risk for nutritional deprivation, the intervention also featured measures such as "nutritional supplementation."[90] Using a mélange of political and psychological terms, the authors claimed that this early intervention was the first step in breaking "the cycle of poverty at the beginning." By giving the children the necessary "conceptual and adaptation tools," this intervention would provide them with future freedom of choice.[91] This project was in effect an early child care enrichment program with an in-home intervention and was explicitly compared to Project Head

Start.[92] The distinctions among different forms of deprivation and between poverty and intellectual disability were blurred beyond recognition. While describing the detrimental effects of the impoverished home life and "meager" maternal interaction that supposedly characterized low-income homes, the researchers offered no discussion of the impact of race beyond mentioning that the program exclusively targeted African American children.

These three interventions demonstrate how different forms of deprivation became the framework by which to interpret "mild mental retardation" and served as the target for expert intervention. Although "cultural deprivation" was used to describe children from low-income families who were seen as "mildly mentally retarded," these interventions focused on providing adequate sensory stimulation and changing the home environment created by mothers. While the first intervention targeted Euro-American children from low-income homes, the programs in Milwaukee and Washington, D.C., targeted solely black children in inner-city neighborhoods, reflecting a change that had occurred from the late 1950s to the mid-1960s. Whereas "cultural deprivation" was first used to describe low-income rural Euro-American families, particularly in the Appalachian region, it soon became synonymous with the urban black poor. Accordingly, this group became the target of interventions designed to prevent or alleviate perceived "mild mental retardation." Yet until the late 1960s, little attention was given to the fact that the category "mild mental retardation" was applied primarily to African American children. Rather, most articles avoided any discussion of race. Some researchers noted that African American children were chosen as subjects for intervention for reasons of convenience and availability, while others focused on socioeconomic factors such as "poverty" or life in an "inner-city" environment—terms that became euphemisms for race.

Intervention or Resegregation?

By the late 1960s, however, race could no longer be ignored. In 1967, Julius Hobson, an African American civil rights activist, filed a lawsuit against Carl Hansen, superintendent of the Washington, D.C., public school system.[93] Prompted by scholastic testing that led to the exclusion of his ten-year-old daughter from the college preparatory track at her school, Hobson sought to end to what he viewed as the systematic denial of educational opportunities to African American children by means of ability grouping and tracking along with blatant inequalities in the allocation of resources.

Tracking had been in place in the Washington, D.C., schools since 1956, when Hansen, the system's associate superintendent at the time, instituted an extensive reform of high school education designed to reduce academic heterogeneity within each classroom. This system was set in place soon after the District of Columbia schools were desegregated. The 1954 *Brown v. Board of Education* decision was rapidly implemented in the District, bringing children from different racial, economic, and scholastic backgrounds into the same classrooms. The tracking system Hansen devised necessitated that each high school student be placed on one of four tracks: basic, general, college preparatory, and honors. The basic track was targeted at children who scored less than seventy-five on IQ tests—the contemporary definition of "mentally retarded." Hansen was a staunch supporter of desegregation, traveling across the country to lecture on the city's perceived successful desegregation of its schools, and he insisted that the tracking system was about ability rather than race.[94] At a time when inner-city school districts faced the challenges not only of desegregation but also of a steady of influx of poor African American families from the rural South, Washington's high school students improved their scores on standardized tests, sending a higher proportion of black students to colleges than any of the nation's other urban school systems.[95] Thus, while some critics had questioned the tracking system in the late 1950s, Hansen's approach was widely supported until the middle of the following decade. In fact, when Hobson attempted to organize a school boycott in 1967 to protest the tracking system, he received little support from the black community; many parents were pleased with Hansen, his methods, and perhaps most significantly, his results.

Hobson v. Hansen was groundbreaking in that it called attention to the racial implications of the tracking system. Hobson argued that the intelligence tests that served as the basis for grouping had been standardized according to results from Euro-American children and thus were culturally biased. Furthermore, he argued, they inaccurately predicted academic success for children from low-income or African American homes. Judge J. Skelly Wright of the Washington, D.C., Court of Appeals excoriated the city's tracking system.[96] The tracking closely corresponded with race, creating de facto segregated classes in desegregated schools and was therefore found to be discriminatory and unconstitutional. Wright's verdict was the first of many that addressed the question of scholastic tracking and its correspondence with race, ethnicity, and economic status and called public and professional attention to the overdiagnosis of African American children as "mentally retarded." The case generated much public attention and mixed responses. Some African American activists and parents viewed the verdict as a triumph over de facto segregation.[97] Others, such African American journalist William Raspberry, who went on to win a Pulitzer Prize, worried about the impact of a ruling that might abolish special education for children who needed these services. He cited his conversation with a mother whose young daughter had been making steady progress on a slow track and had been transferred to a regular class. Struggling with her studies, the child now often returned home in tears.[98] Some white parents withdrew their children from public schools rather than have them sit in the same classrooms as students who had previously been relegated to slow tracks. Some teachers supported this change: One teacher commented candidly that the "security" children might have felt in a basic track class was useless if they did not receive an adequate education.[99] Because the Washington Board of Education refused to appeal Judge Wright's decision, Hansen resigned and appealed personally, though his effort failed. The District of Columbia's school tracking system was eliminated.[100]

In 1968, Lloyd Dunn, past president of the Council for Exceptional Children, an international professional organization dedicated to serving the needs of both disabled and gifted children, published an influential article, "Special Education for the Mildly Retarded—Is Much of It Justifiable?" This article is often credited as the first to call attention to the overrepresentation of children from minority ethnicities and from "nonmiddle-class environments" in special education.[101] Dunn stated baldly, "We must stop labeling these deprived children as mentally retarded. . . . [W]e must stop segregating them by placing them into our allegedly special programs."[102] Dunn cited the *Hobson v. Hansen* verdict and accurately predicted that additional lawsuits would follow. He added that had he been a "Negro from the slums or a disadvantaged parent," he too would have gone to the courts "before allowing the schools to label my child as 'mentally retarded' and place him in a 'self contained special school or class.'"[103]

Dunn criticized the current trend toward "special" separate classes for children, mainly minority and low-income, diagnosed as "retarded." Although he rejected the label "mentally retarded," Dunn clearly embraced the cultural deprivation approach. Arguing that special education would continue to be "a sham of dreams unless we immerse ourselves into the total environment of our children from inadequate homes and backgrounds and insist on a comprehensive ecological push," Dunn held that education was only part of the necessary intervention. Thus, Dunn called for interventions in the home lives of low-income and minority children to alleviate perceived deprivation—without, however, labeling them "mentally retarded" and placing them in de facto segregated classrooms. Dunn's critique was widely cited, and many heeded his call for policymakers and educators to be aware of the "serious educational and civil rights issues" that arose from special education class placement.[104]

The President's Panel on Mental Retardation's 1969 conference on "Problems of Education of Children in the Inner City" addressed these concerns. Although the conference title made no mention of intellectual disability, it was clearly assumed that the education of inner-city children was a problem to be addressed by experts in "mental retardation." The report's introduction explained the ties between these two seemingly unrelated fields. The mass migration of African American families from the rural South to inner cities in the 1950s and 1960 had brought many low-income African American children into inner-city schools. These children scored "low enough on individual tests of intelligence to be classified as mentally retarded," but the "production of so many functionally retarded children by our society raised disturbing questions." The conference's final report, decorated with large, glossy pictures of children from different racial and ethnic backgrounds, was provocatively titled *The Six-Hour Retarded Child.* Below a photo of a young African American child were the words, "We now have what may be called a 6-hour retarded child—retarded from 9 to 3, 5 days a week, solely on the basis of an IQ, without regards to his adaptive behavior, which may be exceptionally adaptive to the situation and community in which he lives."[105] The conference's ninety-two participants, who the report repeatedly emphasized included white, African American, and Hispanic researchers, educators, and inner-city residents, based their discussions mainly on papers by Columbia University education professor Edmund Gordon; Wilson C. Riles, associate superintendent and chief of compensatory education at the California State Department of Education; and James O. Miller, director of the National Laboratory on Early Childhood Education in Urbana, Illinois. Both Gordon and Riles were African Americans. Excerpts from these three papers also appeared in the conference report.

The report included seven recommendations, the first of which was to "provide early childhood stimulation, education, and evaluation as part of the continuum of public education."[106] Providing sensory experiences was seen as a powerful means of preventing future mental retardation. The fourth recommendation was for a reexamination of the current system of intelligence testing and classification and, in particular, withholding a diagnosis of "retardation" until attempts at "remediation" had been made. The report cited Riles's claim that "if the child—black or white or brown—is not very tidy, clothes a little tattered, if he is inarticulate in the English language, many teachers' first reaction is that the child must be mentally retarded." James Allen, New York State commissioner of education and a staunch supporter of desegregation, went so far as to suggest that "mental retardation" was no longer a concept of value for educators, asking whether it could be replaced by a new concept of education for children with special needs.

Riles was one of the most vocal critics of the overrepresentation of African American students in special education classes. In his conference presentation, he noted that "the rate of placement of Spanish surname children in special education is about three times higher than for Anglo children; the Negro rate is close to four times higher than the Anglo rate." He added that the "higher rate of mental retardation in poverty areas may be due to the organic damage resulting from lack of adequate health care, dietary deficiencies, etc." Still, he asked, "to what extent are children classified as mentally retarded when the true nature of their learning disabilities stems from environmental factors?" In California, educators were reexamining their classification criteria "to see if language difficulties, deprivation of experiences, and deviation from the majority's culture and value system" had shaped the diagnosis of "mental retardation." In some school districts, Riles reported, new efforts were being made to reclassify "borderline mentally retarded" children as eligible for compensatory education rather than placement in a special education class. This change would result in more intensive preparatory training for these children, who might later rejoin mainstream education. He cited another project in which preschool children originally diagnosed as "mentally retarded" were placed in regular kindergarten classes after completing a compensatory preschool program.[107] Riles clearly criticized the use of the "mentally retarded" category and was wary of the political significance of the overrepresentation of African American and Hispanic children in special education classes. At the same time, he seemed to strongly support theories of cultural deprivation, citing a lack of early experiences and of shared cultural values as causing scholastic disadvantage.

In 1971, Riles was elected California's superintendent of public instruction, defeating Maxwell Rafferty, the conservative white incumbent. A prominent African American cognizant of racial inequalities in education, Riles must have been surprised when he was named as the main defendant, alongside the education board members, in a class-action lawsuit filed late in the year with the support of the National Association for the Advancement of Colored People (NAACP). The case, *Larry P. v. Riles*, disputed the placement of African American students in classes for the "mentally retarded" on the basis of contested testing procedures. In 1975, before the suit was resolved in favor of the plaintiffs four years later, a moratorium was imposed on the use of intelligence tests for class placement of the state's African American schoolchildren.[108] The American Psychological Association refrained from filing an amicus brief in this extremely controversial case, citing a lack of scientific consensus regarding the validity of the intelligence tests in question.[109] Riles was the only defendant to appeal the 1979 decision, and in 1984, the court reversed the earlier verdict that the defendants' actions demonstrated an "unlawful segregative intent" and was a form of willful discrimination against the plaintiffs.[110] The 1984 verdict cited Riles's 1969 statement regarding the need for a reexamination of the diagnosis of children as "retarded" as evidence that he had not engaged in active discrimination against African Americans.[111] Throughout his career, Riles maintained that if the scholastic tests were discriminatory, they discriminated by socioeconomic status and not by race, and he testified that the worst scores were recorded by "isolated, disadvantaged people of the Appalachia," who were "the purest Anglo Saxon stock in the country."[112]

Riles's career was not derailed by this lawsuit. He enjoyed considerable support from both his supervisors and his community, and as superintendent, he was highly esteemed. When a technicality threatened to prevent him from running for reelection in 1973, he received overwhelming support, including a two-page *Los Angeles Sentinel* article, "Join the Fight to Save Wilson Riles," that made no reference to the ongoing lawsuit. Riles won reelection twice and remained in office until 1983, when he turned to private educational consulting. As superintendent, he strongly advocated equal educational opportunities and continued to defend the judicious use of intelligence testing, refusing to entirely reject a form of testing simply because it was at times misused.[113] The African American press supported Riles and his work, and in 1974, *Ebony* chose him as one of the one hundred most influential African Americans.[114] Riles received numerous honors for his contributions to education, including seven honorary doctorates and the NAACP's Spingarn medal, whose previous recipients had included Martin Luther King Jr. and the assassinated civil rights activist Medgar Evers. Riles received this award in 1973, a year after the NAACP had supported the suit that named Riles as a defendant.[115] Riles and the lawsuit to which he will forever be tied exemplify the contentious nature of debates over placement and intelligence testing in the mid-1970s.

Conclusion

The inclusive criteria of the 1961 *AAMD Manual*, which set the cutoff for mental retardation at one standard deviation below the mean IQ, enabled the diagnosis of a large group of individuals, most of them children, as "mildly mentally retarded."[116] In 1973, the classification was revised, moving the cutoff to two standard deviations below the mean, a decision that reflected at least in part attempts by researchers in the field of intellectual disabilities to reduce the overrepresentation of children from racial minorities.[117] Although the number of children diagnosed as intellectually disabled has declined further since 1974, African American children continue to have a disproportionate rate of placement in separate "special education" classes.[118]

In 1975, Congress passed the Education for All Handicapped Children Act, which ensured that all children, regardless of disability status, would have access to education. Later modified and renamed the Individuals with Disabilities Education Act (IDEA), the law provided for a "free and appropriate education" in the "least restrictive environment." This principle favors mainstreaming and an approach based on the provision of supportive services rather than placement in either general or "special" classes. The 1997 amendment to the law required that states report the number of children receiving services under IDEA, broken down according to race and disability status, to enable federal monitoring of disproportionality. Any state found to engage in such disproportionate identification would need to revise its placement policies.[119]

In the early and mid-1960s, "mild mental retardation" became a loose term, associated with poverty and deprivation and used mainly to describe African American and other minority children from low-income homes. Researchers slowly became aware that this designation, as psychologist Henry Leland stated in 1970, was "first and foremost a political term used to categorize large numbers of individuals."[120]

The creation of the highly political category "mild mental retardation" was made possible by its reliance on deprivation as an etiological theory. As intellectual disability became associated with poverty and perceived deprivation, the interventions designed to prevent or alleviate this disability pathologized the home life and parenting styles of low-income African American families. Entire families could be viewed as "retarded." Any stereotype of poverty—from the presence of rodents to the absence of furniture—could be reinterpreted as a pathogenic form of deprivation. These perceived characteristics became the target for intervention, which was described as a way to "break the cycle of pathology." Researchers increasingly targeted the home environment and parenting abilities of culturally and linguistically diverse persons from low-income backgrounds rather than calling for an evaluation of the causes of socioeconomic disadvantage.

The creation of the category "mild mental retardation" ostensibly was designed to improve the welfare of children from impoverished areas. Rather than viewing poor children as being constitutionally mentally defective, the deprivation theory of intellectual disability propounded an environmentalist approach to intelligence, thus taking a clear stance in the nature-nurture debate. Politicians, educators, and child health experts argued for the medical necessity of providing educational experiences for children from low-income and minority homes. In this manner, the prevention of intellectual disability provided the scientific rationale for the use of government funding for programs benefiting urban African American families, a funding priority that otherwise would have been seen as controversial and problematic. By avoiding a discussion of race and focusing on the health effects of deprivation and the high social costs of intellectual disability, liberal politicians of the early and mid-1960s could justify funding programs benefiting the "undeserving poor."[121] Portraying an epidemic of "mildly mentally retarded" children of unspecified race and ethnicity caused by potentially preventable deprivation provided the Kennedy and later Johnson administrations with ammunition to further their social interventions, especially during the War on Poverty. Social concerns piggybacked on increased public interest in intellectual disability and benefited from its positive image, acquired through media depictions of normative white families struggling to raise disabled children. The growing public support for measures to assist children with disabilities could thus be mobilized to promote a riskier and less popular political agenda—the provision of equal educational opportunities for children from low-income and minority homes.

Yet the widely embraced diagnosis of "mild mental retardation" caused by deprivation has another side: the resulting overdiagnosis of African American children and their placement in special education classes or on slower tracks. These separate classes denied children access to a wide range of educational opportunities, from learning in an academically and racially heterogeneous classroom to participating in advanced courses that would have better prepared these students for a college education. The creation of the "mild mental retardation" category enabled the diagnosis of a large proportion of African American children as intellectually disabled. As desegregation brought more African American children from diverse educational backgrounds into hitherto racially and socioeconomically homogeneous schools, this diagnosis in effect enabled schools to continue a scientifically sound form of segregation. By conflating cultural deprivation with "mild mental retardation," children's racial and socioeconomic backgrounds served as indicators for diagnoses of intellectual ability or disability. Although no hard data exist on the number of African American children who received this diagnosis in the early and mid-1960s, Dunn estimated in 1968 that between 60 and 80 percent of pupils in the special education system came from minority and low-income families. In the 1960s, therefore, "mild mental retardation" was indeed a tool for resegregation.[122]

Today, African American children are still identified for special education classes at rates double and triple those for Euro-American children.[123] Deprivation is no longer an accepted etiological factor for intellectual disability, which is currently classified through a multidimensional approach. This diagnostic system, last revised by the American Association of Intellectual and Developmental Disabilities (AAIDD) in 2010, is designed to assess the need for different individualized support services. Still, traces of the 1959 manual can be discerned among the "social risk factors for intellectual disability," which include poverty, maternal malnutrition, impaired child-caregiver interaction, and the lack of adequate stimulation, described also as "extreme social deprivation." Having completely disavowed the cultural deprivation approach, the deprivations listed by the AAIDD manual echo maternal, sensory, and nutritional deprivation, the main constituents of the cultural deprivation approach.[124] In this manner, although cultural deprivation lost its respectability in scientific discourse, the term's meaning is still retained, demonstrating the long-lasting effect of theories of deprivation on the field of intellectual disability.

CHAPTER FIVE

Environmental Psychology and the Race Riots

ON A SPRING NIGHT IN 1964, as Catherine Genovese was returning to her New York apartment from her work as a night manager at a bar, she was raped and murdered. Initial reports (later found to be unsubstantiated) indicated that as many as thirty-eight of her neighbors witnessed the attack or heard her screams, and none had called the police or offered their help.[1] The crime itself was gruesome, but what mainly aroused public debate at the time was the fact that it had taken place in the victim's home neighborhood and that none of her neighbors had come to her aid. This attack occurred at a time when the urban environment was seen to be dangerous and threatening. Following Genovese's death, Stanley Milgram and other mental health experts tried to explain how such an attack could have happened. In interviews and articles, these experts analyzed the psyche of inner-city residents, making sense of their perceived detachment and lack of empathy.[2] These attempts to gain psychological insight into Genovese's neighbors' inaction typified current trends in American mental health sciences. The 1960s saw a surge of interest in the environment's role in human development and psychology, and scientists and politicians alike exalted the relations between a healthy environment and a healthy psyche.[3]

Environmental psychology received its impetus from sensory deprivation experiments of the late 1950s and early 1960s. Theories of deprivation provided the intellectual framework for basic tenets of environmental psychology. In the wake of urban riots and their investigation by the National Advisory Commission on Civil Disorders (commonly known as the Kerner Commission after its chair, Illinois governor Otto Kerner), deprivation theory enabled social scientists and psychologists to promote a simultaneously medicalized and highly political understanding of urban violence.

The resurgence of environmentalist approaches to human development in the 1960s led many researchers to attempt to examine, isolate, and quantify the components of the environment that were deemed most crucial to human development and individual psychology. This interest in the environment also reflected a growing concern about the detrimental effects of living in inner cities. As affluent white Americans gradually moved to the suburbs after World War II, inner-city neighborhoods became home to African Americans. In turn, white families abandoned urban neighborhoods in fear of a decrease in property values and quality of life. By the late 1950s, this process, later known as "white flight," had amplified even further, as white Americans fled cities with a growing sense of urgency. The inner city remained home to impoverished minorities, as white Americans ensconced themselves in segregated suburbs.[4]

In the late 1940s and 1950s, the inner-city "slums" that had hastily been left behind served as an inspiration for a film noir genre that provided a vivid and racialized portrayal of urban decadence, including black nightclubs, Turkish baths, and decrepit Chinatowns.[5] As cultural historian Eric Avila has shown, these films, with titles such as *Dark City, City of Fear, The Naked City*, and *Cry of the City*, reflected fears of both urban violence and ethnic Otherness. These fantasies served as the backdrop for the growing public and academic interest in the evils of urbanization. Many white observers believed that overcrowded and dilapidated houses in run-down neighborhoods provided evidence of individual deficiency rather than being the result of poverty and inequality. These decaying urban neighborhoods populated nearly exclusively by low-income African Americans further confirmed many white Americans' deep-seated beliefs of their own racial superiority.[6] The race riots of the 1960s further consolidated the view of inner cities as inherently violent and menacing. These images of violent black inner cities hastened the rise of urban psychology. By 1968, this field of inquiry was so well established that parents and children could play the "cities game," a board game similar to Monopoly developed by *Psychology Today*'s editor, David Popoff. Players could take on the role of the government, "agitators," businessmen, or "slum dwellers."[7]

In the late 1950s and early 1960s, scientists and concerned citizens warned the public of modern life's cost to the natural environment. Pollution, overpopulation, and the indiscriminate use of pesticides became highly contested topics. In 1962, environmentalist and marine biologist Rachel Carson published *Silent Spring*, in which she warned of the devastating effects of pesticides. The book was pivotal in bringing environmental concerns to the center of public debate.[8] Environmental studies referred both to the effects of modernization on the natural environment and to how the modern, urban environment affected individuals. The detrimental effects of urban living on individual psychology became the new front for environmentally minded and politically savvy behavioral scientists. The Group for the Advancement of Psychiatry (GAP) organized a symposium dedicated to the topic of mental health in urban communities, examining questions related to the psychiatric implications of urbanization and social planning.[9] Psychologist Marc Fried, best known for his work on the psychological results of urban renewal programs in Boston, highlighted the similarities between early descriptions of institutionalized children suffering from maternal deprivation and the psychiatric disorders caused by long-lasting social deprivation.[10] A mid-1960s editorial in *Science* cited environmental psychology as the "newest fad" in "Washington and elsewhere." By the early 1970s, environmental psychology showed signs of becoming a mainstream, established discipline. A number of influential books and articles were published on the topic, key researchers in the field wrote their reminiscences of the field's evolution, a graduate program at the City University of New York had been established, and the National Institute of Mental Health (NIMH) funded research projects examining the relationship between the physical environment and mental health.[11] Environmental psychologists focused on the role of crowding, inadequate housing, playgrounds for children, and optimal planning of institutions such as hospitals and prisons. Researchers also turned their attention to topics as diverse as the design of bathrooms to enable privacy within a home and how the behavior of cats could provide insight into human behavior.[12]

Race riots erupted in Harlem in 1964 and soon spread throughout the nation, with an estimated 239 riots occurring between 1964 and 1968.[13] By the late 1960s, the hope and optimism that had characterized the early supporters of the civil rights movement had been replaced by fear and what was later termed the "white backlash."[14]

For many environmental psychologists, the riots and their drastic impact on American society led to a shift in research priorities. By the mid-1960s, researchers turned their attention to the role slum conditions might play in the genesis of urban violence. Animal studies had an important role in the development of environmental psychology, and environmental scholars cited seminal works such as those by John B. Calhoun on Norway rats in crowded conditions; these studies were also reproduced in edited volumes on urban studies and environmental psychology. Calhoun, an animal ecologist at the NIMH, spent decades working with rats raised in severely crowded conditions. His studies examined the psychological and physiological pathologies caused by life in extremely crowded conditions, documenting a rise in violence and aggression, abnormal sexual behavior, a loss of maternal behavior, infanticide and even cannibalism. He termed this disintegration of social behavior the "behavioral sink." Using moralizing anthropomorphic descriptions to portray the rats' behavior, Calhoun viewed his work on animals as almost directly applicable to humans.[15] Calhoun cooperated with Menninger-trained community mental health expert Leonard Duhl to organize an interdisciplinary seminar on the impact of the physical environment on behavior. Its proceedings, including Calhoun's research, were later published in Duhl's edited volume, *The Urban Condition*, which Duhl later described as the first book to examine health and cities in a systemic and ecological way.[16] Throughout the 1960s and early 1970s, researchers examined the implications of Calhoun's work on social psychology through ambitious attempts to directly correlate animal findings with human behavior. In 1972, three sociologists relied on Calhoun's animal studies in their examination of the effects of population density on social pathology. Yet they noted that when using "animal studies as a guide," it was unclear what effects to look for in humans, as "density appears to affect different species in different ways." They explained how they planned to translate Calhoun's findings on animals to indexes meaningful in humans. For example, they used the number of minor recipients of public assistance as a surrogate marker for what Calhoun and other animal researchers had described as "ineffectual care of the young."[17]

Popular Science and Environmental Psychology

Sensory deprivation provided the theoretical basis that enabled scientists of different backgrounds and training to engage with questions concerning the role of the environment in shaping individual psychology. French-born bacteriologist René Dubos, working at the Rockefeller Institute for Medical Research (which became Rockefeller University in 1965), turned in the 1960s to issues of environment and particularly pollution. He attained international fame as an important thinker on the natural environment, and his work was made accessible to a wide audience through articles in popular magazines such as in *Psychology Today*.[18] A prolific writer and sought-after speaker and later recipient of the Pulitzer Prize, Dubos was said to have given an average of forty lectures a year, most of them at public rather than academic venues.[19] His 1965 *Man Adapting*, written for a wide audience, established Dubos as a leading expert in environmental research. Dubos referred extensively to early sensory deprivation research, citing research on animals and humans including the experiments of psychologist Donald Hebb. On the basis of these findings, Dubos argued that monotony was not only "boring" but could become an "etiological agent for various types of mental disorders."[20] Thus, Dubos effectively expanded the theory of sensory deprivation to include less extreme and far more mundane conditions. He relied on sensory deprivation experiments to argue that the "very structure of the mind is determined by environmental stimuli," supporting an environmental approach to the determinants of intelligence.[21]

An even more expansive approach to the etiological role of deprivation was articulated in Dubos's 1968 article, "The Crisis of Man in His Environment." Dubos argued that deprivation, social or biological, early in life was responsible for irreversible damage to the learning ability of members of underprivileged populations. Children raised in the slums, he contended, did not acquire the necessary stimuli early in life, a deficiency that ultimately limited the "full utilization of their free will."[22] Dubos emphasized the necessity of a stimulating environment for normal human development and warned of the dangers of sensory deprivation.

Other interdisciplinary scholars shared Dubos's approach, including anthropologist Edward T. Hall. The author of a best-selling 1959 book on cross-cultural differences in communication, Hall gained the status of an academic celebrity.[23] Hall's extensive work on interpersonal communications and cultural norms appeared in venues ranging from the *Harvard Business Review* to *Playboy*.[24] Hall's 1966 book for a popular audience, *The Hidden Dimension*, developed a unique theory of proxemics—"man's use of space as a specialized elaboration of culture."[25] Sensory deprivation experiments provided Hall with the theoretical basis to explain phenomena as diverse as driving in a car through a monotonous landscape and the dangers of living in inadequate housing without a window view.[26] Drawing on descriptions of animal experiments, Hall argued that "caged animals become stupid, which is a very heavy price to pay for a super filing system!" Such animal crowding was analogized to the crowded housing projects, as Hall specifically referred to dangerous living conditions in Harlem. Comparing caged animals to inner-city residents, he asked pointedly, "How far can we afford to travel down the road of sensory deprivation in order to file people away?"[27] He relied on sensory deprivation theory to critique crowded, dilapidated housing conditions. Describing apartments with no window views located in monotonous, sprawling concrete neighborhoods, Hall argued that sensory deprivation was an inherent risk of living in decaying neighborhoods. His use of animal experiments was designed to highlight the dangers of urban living and represented a call to take environmental psychology into account in urban design.

Thus, these two popular scientists relied on sensory deprivation theory to provide a scientific basis for their speculations about the relations between the environment and individual psychology. Stretching the limits of the theory, both men attempted to present common everyday phenomena as on the same spectrum as the extreme conditions of experimental sensory deprivation. In so doing, they enlisted the prestige of sensory deprivation to warn of the dangers of the inner city and highlight the urgency of urban reform.

Other, lesser-known scientists joined Dubos and Hall in turning away from their usual academic pursuits to grapple with the urban environment's role in mental health. While some ventured into this field from somewhat related disciplines such as geography or architecture, others indeed were a long way from home. Albert E. Parr, former director and senior scientist at the American Museum of Natural History and a researcher on oceanography and marine biology, published a number of articles on the relationship between the urban environment and individual mental health.[28] He relied on sensory deprivation experiments to elaborate his approach to environmental studies. After citing the work of laboratory researchers on the effects of a completely "monotonous" environment, Parr argued that he had seen "nothing to suggest that urban monotony and experimental monotony should differ in anything but degree." Thus, Parr paralleled urban and laboratory conditions and the effects of sensory deprivation and metropolitan living conditions.[29] In a different article, he argued that sensory deprivation experiments indicated the need to examine the correlation between environmental diversity (ranging from "normal" to the "monotony" of an urban environment) and intellectual performance. The extreme conditions of sensory deprivation experiments were seen as on a clear continuum with "urban monotony."[30] Although untrained in the field of mental health, Parr speculated about the influence of dilapidated urban housing on individual psychology, highlighting the ubiquitousness of concerns regarding the psychological effects of inner cities.

Environmental psychologists relied on creative interpretations of sensory deprivation theories to explain diverse cultural phenomena. One researcher examined how housing effected marital interactions in light of ongoing urbanization and the lack of large open spaces. "Wandering in meadows, fishing in pleasant streams," he lamented, were activities of yore. In the urban environment, spouses grew bored with each other as a symptom of sensory deprivation induced by their unstimulating home environments. Women, he speculated, carried out home improvements to create more stimulating environments and consequently ward off psychological discontent. Nearly one-fifth of all Americans lived in environments "almost entirely devoid of any kind of esthetic or psychological stimulation."[31]

These interdisciplinary interpretations of sensory deprivation were common. At a conference on housing, one psychiatrist cited the works of John Bowlby and studies on marasmus to emphasize the role of the home environment in providing sufficient stimulation.[32] Surprisingly perhaps, suburban life was not described as depriving. In 1963, feminist Betty Friedan published her indictment of the life of the suburban homemaker, *The Feminine Mystique*.[33] Although she emphasized the boredom and monotony of suburban life and domestic chores, Friedan made no reference to sensory deprivation or to the role of the physical environment. Relying on the work of child psychologist Bruno Bettelheim, who had used concentration camp imagery to describe why certain children's homes were destructive to their psyches, Friedan compared suburban homes to "comfortable concentration camps." Familiar with recent developments in American psychology, Friedan clearly did not shy away from difficult imagery.[34] Yet in the 1960s, critics of repressive suburban American lives did not align themselves with environmental psychology and did not compare suburban living to a form of sensory deprivation, a comparison reserved for inner-city homes.[35]

This focus on the pathogenic role of the crowded urban environment can be tied to the emerging field of "ekistics." The term, coined by Greek architect and urban planner Constantinos Doxiadis in 1942, referred to the science of human settlements and reflected the growing interest in a humanist approach to urban development. This approach was embraced by the Ford Foundation, which supported Doxiadis's work and funded a new journal, *Ekistics*, and an annual conference known as the Delos Symposium. Among the participants of the first conference was Leonard Duhl, who had a long-standing interest in community mental health and the impact of the environment on individual psychology.[36]

René Dubos's work profoundly influenced the development of the field of ekistics, and his writings were cited extensively by researchers from diverse disciplinary backgrounds. In fact, Doxiadis, commonly seen as the father of the field, relied on Dubos's definitions of health in the major introductory text to the field. Dubos's writings—the reflections of an esteemed scientist writing for a popular audience—influenced the development of this new discipline.[37]

An interest in the pathology caused urban life led environmental psychologists to take a second look at sensory deprivation experiments, drawing parallels between the extreme laboratory conditions and the daily reality of urban living. Clark University environmental psychologist Joachim Wohlwill relied heavily on sensory deprivation experiments. Editing a 1964 issue of the *Journal of Social Issues* dedicated to "man's response to the physical environment," Wohlwill brought together scientists from diverse backgrounds. The contributors included Albert Parr, John Calhoun, psychologists, sociologists, an architect, geographers, and a consultant to the government described as a specialist in the field of "clothing, housing and economic development."[38] The contributors repeatedly referred to sensory deprivation research. Geographer Robert Kates hailed Dubos for calling attention to "the stimulus properties of the environment"—that is, the ability of a certain environment to provide adequate sensory stimulation.[39] Psychologist Robert Sommer attributed current interest in the physical environment as a variable in psychological research to the early sensory deprivation experiments carried out by Hebb and his colleagues.[40] Many of the studies focused on the role of environmental stimulation, attempting to identify what amount and types of external stimuli were necessary for optimal development and psychological well-being. In this manner, environmental psychologists tied sensory deprivation experiments, which attempted to isolate different forms of stimulation through the use of devices such as goggles, gloves, earmuffs, and liquid food, to observations of individuals in their home environments.

These studies were mainly impressionistic. No clear criteria for evaluating the adequacy of environmental stimulation were proposed, nor were attempts made to provide a method of analyzing the effects of this stimulation. Yet all of the scholars agreed that stimulation or the lack thereof within the urban home environment had effects similar to, if less extreme than, those observed in the sensory deprivation experiments. Wohlwill later published "The Emerging Discipline of Environmental Psychology" in the widely circulated *American Psychologist*, again relying heavily on sensory deprivation experiments.[41] While much research has been carried out on understimulation, he argued, little had been done on the dangers of overstimulation. "We are better informed of the psychological hazards of extended stays in the antarctic," he argued, "than in megalopolis." The oft-cited experiments in sensory deprivation and their popular tropes, such as Arctic travel, provided the theoretical framework by which to interpret a broadening spectrum of phenomena as relevant to environmental psychology.

The Environment in Psychiatry and Beyond

Alongside the rise of environmental psychology, the environment gained recognition as an important factor in mainstream, individual psychiatry. Clinicians became more cognizant of the role of the environment in their patients' psychic makeup. Representative of this trend was psychiatrist and psychoanalyst Harold Searles, who in 1960 published his first monograph, *The Nonhuman Environment in Normal Development and in Schizophrenia*. Searles lamented the disregard with which psychiatry continued to view what he termed the "nonhuman environment" despite growing evidence of its importance. Psychiatrists, he argued, often erred in focusing solely on interpersonal relationships.[42] In arguing for the importance of the environment, he relied on both experiments in sensory deprivation and descriptions of maternal deprivation, such as René Spitz's early work. These maternal deprivation studies, Searles argued, provided information about the lack of "nonhuman environmental stimuli" rather than a lack of mothering; with this statement, he took a clear stance in the debate over the uniqueness of maternal deprivation.[43] Citing the findings of major studies in sensory deprivation research, Searles argued that the resulting hallucinations occurred "as if to fill the void caused by the experimentally induced sensory deprivation." In healthy subjects, this void was experimentally induced through sensory deprivation, which led them to hallucinate. Persons with schizophrenia, Searles argued, perceived their world to be so "unpeopled and otherwise bleak"—so sensorily deprived—that they projected hallucinations into this void to fill their empty lives.[44] Thus, Searles used sensory deprivation as a framework for understanding psychoses and their relation to the external environment, a theme that continued in Searles's later publications.[45] Psychiatrists referred to the role of sensory deprivation in understanding their patients' relations to the environment while retaining a focus on individual psychology. Some psychoanalysts even highlighted the similarities between experiments in sensory deprivation and the analytic hour, in which the "quiet of the analyst's office, the patient's supine position, his inability to see the analyst and the absence of everyday verbal response" induced regression and assisted in the therapeutic process.[46] Influenced by the rise of environmental psychology, mainstream American mental health experts in the 1960s gradually acknowledged the importance of the environment in understanding the workings of the individual psyche.

From Crowding to Riots

Many mental health experts believed that crowded urban environments caused a unique psychopathology. Often basing their works on Calhoun's animal studies, researchers attempted to develop human models to examine the psychological effects of environmental crowding. Sensory deprivation theory was used in this interpretation in two opposing ways. While some researchers interpreted crowding as at the opposite pole from sensory deprivation, constituting a form of environmental overstimulation, others viewed the crowded environment as a form of deprivation.[47] Some authors specifically referred to the difficulty of controlling for crowding and other forms of deprivation, thus demonstrating that crowding and deprivation were seen to be so close as to be confounders.[48]

The detrimental effects of crowding and the psychological implications of housing were also pressing federal concerns. Social worker and public policy researcher Alvin Schorr, at the time on the research staff of the Social Security Administration, was assigned to evaluate the role of housing policies in targeting poverty. This evaluation sought to propose a housing policy that would aid in the larger goal of eradicating poverty.[49] Schorr's 1963 report, *Slums and Social Insecurity*, included an extensive evaluation of the psychological aspects of housing conditions, perhaps reflecting Schorr's early training as a social worker. He found that although crowding was not the single or major element in producing the "culture of poverty," it combined with other deprivations to shape the "slum dweller."[50] While crowding per se served as a point of departure for many researchers, these works were soon translated into the field of political violence—in particular, analyses of the urban riots of the 1960s.

The Kerner Commission and Theories of Mental Health

Although major race riots had occurred since the early twentieth century, the 1960s saw an escalation in both the frequency and the violence of these riots, with higher death tolls than ever before. In July 1964, violence erupted in Harlem following the shooting of an African American teenager by a white off-duty police officer. Six days of rioting by an estimated eight thousand participants in Harlem and then in another African American community, Bedford-Stuyvesant, led to one death, hundreds of injuries, and hundreds of arrests. This was just the beginning.[51] That summer also saw riots in numerous other cities, including Rochester, New York; Philadelphia; and Jersey City, New Jersey. The following year, five days of riots in Watts, a nearly entirely African American neighborhood in Los Angeles, left thirty-four people dead.[52] California governor Edmund G. Brown Sr. appointed a commission to examine the cause of the riots and develop recommendations for change. Chaired by John McCone, former head of the Central Intelligence Agency, this commission was later criticized for emphasizing the criminal rather than political aspects of the riots. Downplaying the number of participants and highlighting their criminal backgrounds and lack of education, the report attempted to portray the riots as an outburst of criminal activity rather than an event of political significance. This approach blamed the rioters rather than the societal conditions that led to the outbreak of urban violence.[53] Many activists, scholars, and politicians attempted to explain the causes of the riots and propose different solutions, and during the Johnson administration alone, thirteen different municipal and state commissions were initiated to evaluate the riots. Yet the McCone Commission was the most extensive effort to address these questions until President Lyndon Baines Johnson initiated a national evaluation.[54]

The 1967 Detroit riot was the era's most destructive and violent race riot. When the state police and National Guard failed to regain control of the city, President Johnson sent in thousands of paratroopers. Resulting in the deaths of forty-three people, including thirty-three African Americans, injuries to two thousand people, and seven thousand arrests, the riot left an indelible imprint on the city's race relations.[55] With support for the Johnson administration already faltering, the president was forced to act quickly. Five days after the violence in Detroit had erupted, Johnson appointed the National Advisory Commission on Civil Disorders, headed by Illinois governor Otto Kerner. The Kerner Commission was charged with investigating the nationwide riots, determining what had caused them, and making recommendations for preventing further outbreaks of violence.[56] A bipartisan commission, it consisted of eleven members, two of whom were black: Massachusetts senator Edward Brooke and NAACP director Roy Wilkins. The most outspoken liberal was New York City mayor John Lindsay, who served as the commission's vice chair; his views were balanced by those of conservative businessman Charles B. "Tex" Thornton. The commission

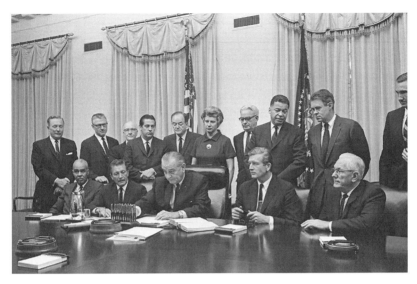

Meeting of the National Advisory Commission on Civil Disorders, 1967. Photo by Yoichi Okamoto. Courtesy of Lyndon Baines Johnson Library and Museum, Austin, Texas.

conducted hearings behind closed doors, solicited expert testimony, and commissioned research groups to examine data on the riots and their participants. NIMH social psychologist Robert Shellow was appointed research director. Shellow, at the time a relatively obscure psychologist, later learned that better-known psychologists had turned down this position, concerned about involvement in a commission that would "whitewash" America's pressing racial problems.[57] He set up a task force of six social scientists to serve as the commission's in-house research team. Large-scale research projects were contracted by the commission or funded by other federal agencies, such as the NIMH. Shellow's team worked tirelessly, examining more than fifteen thousand pages of raw data, including police and fire department logs and witness testimonies about the riots.[58] The commission also relied on psychiatric consultants, including African American psychiatrist and psychoanalyst Charles Pinderhughes, who examined the workings of the rioters' psyches.

Pinderhughes had a long-standing interest in the psychological factors that contributed to urban violence. He emphasized the interrelations between social and medical pathology, urging his colleagues to "employ descriptive medical terminology rather than terms for social pathology" and thus transforming normative social standards into medical norms.[59] Pinderhughes provided the commission with background material on the psychological meanings of protest and prepared a report comparing the psychology of adolescents who participated in peaceful protests with the psychology of those who took part in urban rioting.[60] He espoused psychodynamic interpretations of urban violence, many of which viewed the power relations between whites and African Americans as comparable to those of parents and children.[61] Not shying away from disturbing interpretations, he suggested that African Americans' "brown coloring has reinforced the tendency to link in our unconscious minds images of colored persons with images of body products and body processes which must be excluded from social circumstances."[62]

Yet alongside these psychodynamic interpretations, Pinderhughes was interested in the role of the environment and how it influenced individual psychology. In crowded quarters, an adult ego "has a task more comparable with the ego of children," particularly if "family and ethnic" organization do not provide adequate support. Crowding led to an increase in the environmental stimuli that had to be mastered, while "rivalry for objects, service and supplies" and struggles for control were common. Increased density together with a "weakened family and group structure" had a "devastating" effect on mental health. A riot, Pinderhughes argued, was an "epidemic form of disruptive activity which is on-going otherwise in endemic form," such as vandalism.[63] Pinderhughes and a colleague, psychiatrist Herbert Levine, interviewed young male rioters and determined that riots "grew out of and further stimulated pregenital psychology." In contrast, nonviolent protests "stimulated in adolescents a more mature form of genital level psychology."[64] Thus both psychoanalysis and urban psychology informed Pinderhughes's interpretation of the causes of urban violence.

Shellow, political scientist David Boesel, psychologist David Sears, and sociologists Gary Marx and Louis Goldberg prepared a report, "The Harvest of American Racism," that relied on social and political theory to evaluate riots in twenty-three cities, portraying the urban violence as a rebellion against white racism.[65] Depicting rioters as political activists, the report highlighted the responsibility of white American society and of the police in particular. Increasing taxes and developing multibillion-dollar programs to repair urban slums were proposed as necessary to prevent further rioting. This radical document was rejected by the commission, and Shellow and his coauthors were promptly fired, along with 120 staff members. The official reason for this personnel change was funding considerations. Unexpectedly, the work of these social scientists and psychologists had offered a clearly political interpretation of the causes of the riots rather than a depoliticization based on neutral, professional discourse.

Recent scholars who have examined the use of mental health disciplines to explain the outbreak of urban violence in the 1960s have focused on how this professional discourse effectively medicalized and depoliticized the riots.[66] Psychiatrist and cultural critic Jonathan Metzl has argued that the "protest psychosis" became a diagnosis by which to explain the violent and seemingly erratic behavior of "angry black men." Rather than a political statement, Metzl shows, these riots were seen as outbursts resulting from schizophrenia, the diagnosis of which gradually changed to include characteristics such as anger, violence, and suspicion.[67]

One egregious example of such medicalized depoliticization is a 1967 letter to the editor of the *Journal of the American Medical Association.* Penned by psychiatrist Frank Ervin and neurosurgeons Vernon Mark and William Sweet, its title was unmistakable: "Role of Brain Disease in Riots and Urban Violence." The obvious focus on the role of poverty, unemployment, and inadequate education, the three physicians suggested, "may have blinded us to the more subtle role of other possible factors, including brain dysfunction." "Focal brain lesions," they argued, had a causal role in violent behavior; any evaluation of the riots should examine the clinical features of individuals involved to "pinpoint, diagnose and treat" persons with a "low violence threshold" and thus avert further tragedy.[68] Numerous historians of the Kerner Commission have cited this letter, yet focusing solely on such extreme, biologistic responses leads to a one-sided portrayal of the mental health profession's response to the riots.[69] Theories of deprivation enabled mental health professionals to use their expert knowledge to advance highly political yet still medicalized interpretations of the causes of and remedies for the rioting.

The media closely followed the commission's work.[70] The final report was published in 1968 in paperback, designed for the general public. The black cover featured large white lettering and an orange-red frame.[71] Race relations, the cover seemed to suggest, were on fire. One of the questions implicit in this examination was why violence was erupting in a period in which the government had taken action to combat discrimination and improve the daily lives of African Americans. Interest in environmental psychology converged with current politics to ask what about the ghetto led the urban black poor to riot.

The Kerner Commission's views of the riots relied on theories of environmental psychology, particularly interpretations of the detrimental effects of crowding. Letters to the commission members demonstrate the acceptance of the interrelations between environmental and individual psychology;

a cardiologist portrayed the lack of air-conditioning units in public housing as an important contributing factor to the outbreak of violence. An Illinois Department of Health sanitary engineer described studies of children raised in institutions that he believed indicated that growing up without "facilities which afford an opportunity for personal cleanliness, hygiene and privacy" negatively affected children's IQs. An African American behavioral scientist wrote to President Johnson to urge the appointment of an "urbanologist" to the commission.[72]

Historian Ellen Herman has argued that the Kerner Commission's deliberations and final report demonstrate the cardinal role of theories of individual psychology in the understanding of the urban riots. The views held by mental health experts, Herman has shown, were at times "virtually indistinguishable" from those of liberal-leaning politicians. Psychologists, psychiatrists, and government officials thus conceptualized the goals of governmental intervention in similar terminology derived from behavioral science discourse.[73] The Kerner Commission was informed by experts who relied on psychological interpretations of the riots that drew heavily on concepts of deprivation. Consequently, deprivation-based interpretations framed the interventions recommended by the experts who testified before the commission and influenced the commission's final report. While the use of psychological theories to explain why African Americans participate in riots has been criticized as shifting the focus away from the rioters' political motivations and the structural features of American society that created a frustrated, disenfranchised minority, the use of theories of deprivation was highly political.[74]

While the Kerner Commission drew heavily on theories of environmental psychology, psychologists later cited the Kerner Report's conclusions to lend scientific credibility to their own research. Some psychologists devised experiments to evaluate the Kerner Report's hypotheses. Citing the report's contention that the summer heat contributed to the eruption of violence, for example, one group of researchers examined the effect of elevated temperature on "interpersonal affective responses."[75]

Relative and Social Deprivation

Relative deprivation was the form of deprivation most commonly invoked by the Kerner Commission and its experts as a causal factor in the urban riots. The term was first coined in 1949 to examine how military men perceived their promotion opportunities. Soldiers promoted in the military police, where promotion opportunities were uncommon, compared themselves favorably to their peers who had not been promoted. In contrast, in the Army Air Corps, where many promotion opportunities existed, servicemen who had not been promoted compared themselves unfavorably to the large number of promoted peers and experienced feelings of "relative deprivation," a term used to denote the discrepancy between what one has achieved and what one perceives as one's entitlement.[76] In the 1960s, theories of relative deprivation were used to explain why, despite the absolute improvement in African Americans' living conditions, dissatisfaction and frustration were rampant in urban communities. While absolute living conditions had improved, they remained far below those of middle-class white Americans, ostensibly creating a profound sense of frustration among the urban black community, which was said to be at the base of the violent eruptions.[77]

Many people who testified before the commission mentioned or implied the concept of relative deprivation. Kenneth Clark referred to the "discrepancy between promise and fulfillment" as an important factor in the emergence of urban violence. Secretary of Health, Education, and Welfare John Gardner, the highest-ranking psychologist employed by the federal government, referred to the heightened aspirations that resulted from recent social gains, arguing that the "potential for unrest develops as people make enough gains so that they see the possibility of a better life."[78] Even when the specific term "relative deprivation" was not used, the concept informed experts' views on the causes of the urban riots.

Others reinterpreted previously accepted sociological theories in light of relative deprivation. Seymour Martin Lipset, a sociologist and scholar of American exceptionalism, used the concept of relative deprivation rather anachronistically in his discussion of the "urban ghetto." Both Tocqueville and Marx, Lipset argued, had demonstrated the importance of "relative deprivation" as opposed to "stable objective deprivation" in "producing receptivity for revolution."[79]

Relative deprivation would remain the form of deprivation most closely identified with attempts to explain urban unrest.[80] Yet other interpretations of deprivation were evident throughout the testimonies and reports presented before the Kerner Commission, which often relied on descriptions of phenomena as dissimilar as economic deprivation and sensory deprivation.

The NIMH cooperated fully with the Kerner Commission investigation. At the time, the agency was funding research on the cause of "mass violence," supporting nearly fifty projects to the tune of four million dollars. One project at Brandeis University's Lemberg Center for the Study of Violence sought to predict the outbreak of riots, while other studies analyzed the individual psychology of the rioters.[81] A brief, confidential report, "Toward an Understanding of Mass Violence: Contributions from the Behavioral Sciences," prepared by NIMH staff for the Kerner Commission, referred extensively to deprivation. The report argued that the urban riots were not the "senseless and chaotic expressions of 'mad dogs.'" Rather, these riots resulted from "the intense, complex and inclusive system of deprivation to which Negro-Americans living in our urban ghettos have been subjected."[82] This report proposed a novel form of deprivation, "structural deprivation," as contributing to the riots. This term was used to indicate the manner in which social structure relied on de facto discrimination to exclude African Americans. Structural deprivation "put the Negro in the position of being 'invited' to participate equally in the opportunities of American life but simultaneously blocks his entry by making him unprepared and unfit to do so." This "unfitness" resulted from the "the series of deprivation in education, employment, medical care, housing, sources of satisfaction and self respect, etc. which are reflected pervasively through everyday social, legal and economic practices."[83] Thus, the "deprivation" of public services such as housing and medical care was taken to be equal to psychological forms of deprivation. This report viewed deprivation as the core cause of the conditions that lead to rioting. The structure of modern American society profoundly deprived the urban African American community. Structural, economic, and individual psychological deprivation were viewed equally, illustrating the broad outlines of what NIMH researchers held to be relevant psychiatric environmental factors.

Martin Luther King Jr.

The framework of deprivation and compensation reverberated in the testimonies of speakers from diverse backgrounds. Martin Luther King Jr. warned of the "syndrome of deprivation" rampant in the African American community.[84] The 1964 Nobel Peace Prize recipient, King had completed graduate training in theology prior to becoming a Baptist minister and civil rights warrior. He suggested a compensation program, modeled after the GI Bill, to rectify societal inequalities. "Special measures for the deprived have always been accepted in principle by the United States," he argued, citing child labor laws, social security, unemployment benefits, and benefits for war veterans. Noting the long-standing deprivation of African Americans, King suggested compensation for unpaid wages during the slavery period. Such a "bill of rights for the disadvantaged," he asserted, would have a profound effect on the "basic psychological and motivational transformation of the Negro."[85] For King, rectifying economic deprivation could correct psychological deprivation.

King had made nearly identical statements from the early 1960s. His third book, *Why We Can't Wait,* based on his 1963 letter from the Birmingham jail, recounted the events of the civil rights movement in Alabama in the spring and summer of 1963 and included his argument on behalf of a "bill of rights for the disadvantaged." As in his later testimony before the Kerner Commission, King emphasized the psychological changes that would result from the correction of long-standing deprivations. He further emphasized that this "bill of rights" would benefit the white poor, who "also suffer deprivation and the humiliation of poverty if not of color." [86]

Although King emphasized the perils of economic deprivation, he also referred specifically to psychological aspects of deprivation. In *Why We Can't Wait,* King argued that apart from economic changes, a large-scale "social-work apparatus" would be necessary. Poverty created "emotional disturbances," which in turn led to "antisocial acts." Children were the most "tragic victims," since their "impoverished parents, frantically struggling day by day for food and a place to live," were unable "to create the stable home necessary for the wholesome growth of young minds." King also contended that the "separate culture of poverty in which the half-educated Negro lives" had been further compounded by automation, leading to the loss of unskilled and semiskilled jobs.[87]

In his 1964 Nobel Prize lecture, King decried the "miserable culture of poverty" that affected some forty million Americans. Echoing theories of relative deprivation, King argued that the plight of these impoverished Americans was further compounded by their knowledge that "even though they are perishing on a lonely island of poverty they are surrounded by a vast ocean of material prosperity."[88] Throughout the decade, King reiterated this suggestion of compensating African Americans for centuries of deprivation.[89]

Steeped in the rich oral tradition of black folk preachers, King borrowed ideas and even exact phrases from a wide range of influences, creating a unique synthesis.[90] In his sermons and publications, King often relied on terms, metaphors, and ideas appropriated from mental health discourse. In 1961, he had urged his followers to be psychologically "maladjusted," to embrace nonviolent protest against injustice. As Metzl has argued, King used schizophrenia as a metaphor for the experience of the basic African American experience, which involved choosing between anger and the desire to make the right, nonviolent choice. His 1963 letter from Birmingham jail argued that "segregation distorts the soul and damages the personality," using what historian Daryl Scott has termed "damage imagery" to argue for racial equality.[91] Deprivation was the scientific basis on which King could propose a radical restructuring of American society.

Indeed, African American activists used deprivation terminology to highlight governmental neglect and the need for intervention.[92] Willie Thompson, an African American from Virginia and supporter of the Black Power movement, wrote to Senator William B. Spong to argue forcefully that the race riots were caused by long-standing social injustice. Yet Thompson also lamented the fact that many teachers were "not equipped or qualified to teach those who are educationally and culturally deprived," demonstrating that support for Black Power could coexist with an acceptance of cultural deprivation theory.[93]

Parental Deprivation

The Kerner Commission and its expert consultants also saw parental deprivation as a salient field for understanding the causes of the riots. Reflecting the ongoing debate over the controversial 1965 Moynihan Report, commission members were interested in the prevalence of matriarchal African American families and the lack of masculine role models believed to contribute to the outbreak of urban violence.[94] Since both the rioters and the experts who studied them were predominantly male, images of normative masculinity played a significant role in debates regarding participants' psychological characteristics. New York mayor John Lindsay wanted to know whether rioters had been raised in homes of one or two parents, viewing this as a relevant factor in understanding rioters' background.[95] Representative Clarice Heckert, a Delaware Republican, wrote the commission, berating the government and the welfare system that encouraged the increase in "hopeless matriarchal families." Theories of pathologic family structures were held to be of primary importance in deciphering the causes of riots.[96]

The commission's interest in family structure and parental deprivation reached its apex in November 1967 when three sociologists and anthropologists provided their opinions of the causes of urban violence. Hyman Rodman of Detroit's Merrill Palmer Institute and NIMH researcher Elliot Liebow, a salaried Kerner Commission consultant, were promising junior scholars; John Mogey was chair of the sociology department at Boston University. The three experts examined the "structure of the family in the ghetto and its relationship to civil disorders." Liebow had recently published *Tally's Corner: A Study of Negro Streetcorner Men*, a well-received ethnographic study of black men in the urban ghetto in Washington, D.C. A sympathetic portrayal of the plight of African American men in urban centers, Liebow's study became a classic in anthropology.[97] Liebow presented to the Kerner Commission his understanding of the causes of urban riots, which differed from that of many of his contemporaries. He argued that family patterns among the poor represented an adaption to their "deprived circumstances," not a cause of it. Economic circumstances, particularly unemployment, led to the marginal familial positions of men and to familial instability, female-headed families, and ultimately to the conditions that led to riots. Although Liebow emphasized economic deprivation, particularly unemployment, as the principal causal factor in the outbreak of riots, he still echoed contemporary approaches regarding the pathology of black family structure and the dangers of matriarchy. Furthermore, he argued that economic deprivation led to psychological damage and pathology.[98]

Members of the Kerner Commission asked the three experts to address the relations between fatherlessness and rioting. Although Mogey initially claimed that this relationship was probably complex and indirect, he later speculated that the young rioters came mostly from fatherless families.[99] Fatherless families were directly tied to rioting, he argued, since the presence of fathers helped to preserve a "kin network" that "maintains relations with the church and maintains its respect for the recognized agencies of social control, such as the law courts, the police and the social welfare worker." Mogey speculated that the "absence of a man" led to a "breakdown of internal personal control," particularly among adolescents. As a result, fatherless youth suffered from a loss of respect for religion, social welfare, education, police, and the courts. When such norms were lacking, the group was unable internally to regulate its members' behavior, leading to an increasing need for external control. Thus, the "faulty" family structure was causally tied to the conditions leading to the outbreak of the riots.[100] Accordingly, at the end of his testimony and the ensuing discussion, Mogey suggested that the commission support the "the marital unit, that is, the man and the woman as husband and wife" rather than viewing the two only as parents. Strengthening the marital relationship, Mogey believed, would foster mutual respect, and both partners would ultimately fulfill their expected roles and focus on building family unity.[101]

The Kerner Commission was particularly interested in the possible effectiveness of early educational programs in ameliorating ghetto conditions. Could these interventions ultimately prevent the conditions that had led to rioting? Mogey argued that some mothers were "sociologically unfit for motherhood." In fact, he added, mothers were not always the best people to bring up their children.[102] Liebow, in contrast, emphasized that women, including mothers of young children, had a strong need to take part in the adult world and leave their homes. In some "ghetto" homes, he argued, "the plaster is falling out and most of the utilities don't work, perhaps, but the rooms are immaculate because [women] have spent half of their lives just polishing and cleaning things that don't really need to be cleaned."[103] These mothers, he explained, had nothing else to do at home and were desperate to find meaningful occupation. Congressman and commission member James Corman asked Rodman for his opinions of different legislative initiatives that might require women to find employment to be eligible for different welfare benefits. This initiative, Corman explained, would result in the establishment of nurseries nationwide.[104] Rodman responded that for poor African American children, who were at a scholastic disadvantage, early child care and compensatory education could be useful. Still, Rodman criticized psychologists who attempted to administer compensatory enrichment as early as possible with Head Start and other programs targeted at younger children. Eventually, he quipped, "we may have some of our psychologists who believe strongly in early experience and the importance of stimulation and reinforcement . . . standing right there at the delivery room and one day saying to the other, as soon as you see the head, start."[105] Cultural and maternal deprivation and the necessity of compensatory education were integral to the Kerner Commission's discussion on how to shape the image of a nonrioting citizen.

Sensory Deprivation

Matthew Dumont, a psychiatrist and NIMH consultant, had worked closely with Leonard Duhl, who later described Dumont as one of the greatest American community psychiatrists.[106] In his 1968 book, *The Absurd Healer*, a reflection on the role of the community psychiatrist, Dumont referred extensively to the urban riots. Duhl wrote the preface, and Dumont appended a report he had prepared for the Kerner Commission in which he examined the role of youth groups in African American communities.[107] In a chapter on "The City as Patient," Dumont depicted the city as an organism that suffered from four basic deficits: a deficit in stimulation, a deficit in self-esteem, a deficit in sense of community, and a deficit in sense of environmental mastery. All of these deficits led to the "symptomatology" of urban violence; the riots were a symptom of a "sick" city.

Two of these deficits reflected the prevailing interest in the role of the environment in individual psychology. To address the perceived deficit in stimulation, Dumont first summarized current knowledge of sensory deprivation phenomena. He described sensory deprivation laboratory experiments as well as "clinical situations that mirror" experimental ones. Psychosis following ophthalmological surgery or "kayak angst"—when an Eskimo seal hunter who had spent many hours in a kayak was said to act in a bizarre fashion—were attributed to sensory deprivation. Dumont argued for a "biopsychological hunger for stimulation" as basic as the need for food or water. "And what of the ghetto?," Dumont asked rhetorically. Although it might seem to be stimulating, he argued, it was in fact monotonous and unchanging. While some viewers might erroneously believe that the ghetto had an atmosphere of "intense vitality and violent passion," this viewpoint could be attributed to the outsiders' "anxiety and hysteria." The ghetto residents in fact suffered from a "stimulus deprivation" caused by the "lack of expectation of change." Thus, riots could be seen as a desperately needed "input of stimulation" in a sensorily deprived environment.[108] The race riots were depicted as a direct result of sensory deprivation caused by the urban ghetto.

Dumont's definition of a deficit of environmental mastery further highlighted the importance of environmental psychology theories in his interpretation of the urban riots. To illustrate the importance of relations between the environment and the individual, Dumont recounted how infants quickly learn that they can influence their environment by producing certain sounds or grimaces. The extent to which individuals in their early lives learned to control their environments shaped their psychological development. Individuals who failed to learn to adequately control their environments through their own actions could experience "severe emotional disability." In contrast, children who grew up in environments that they could too strictly control would not learn to master their own impulses and would develop a pathological need to control others.[109] Yet the extent to which children could master their environments was not the only potential source of psychopathology

Dumont identified. Having developed an adequate mastery of the environment in childhood, adults who lived in unresponsive environments could develop feelings of rage. A feeling of control over the environment, Dumont explained, was a "basic psychological need." Yet in the ghetto, "the impoverished Negro" could only "react passively and helplessly to the exploitative or bureaucratic institutions that channel his behavior," experiencing no control over the environment.[110] The acceptable forms of exercising power over the environment in adult life were mainly via political engagement or economic action. Because African Americans were excluded from both arenas, Dumont argued, they found other outlets for establishing their environmental mastery, leading to violent urban uprisings.[111]

Dumont's usage of sensory deprivation and environmental psychology was not designed to depoliticize the urban riots or to depict them as physiological outbursts inevitably resulting from certain environmental inputs. His analysis was highly political. "Mental health is freedom," he argued. For sufferers of neuroses, this freedom was "restricted by the internal constraints of repetition-compulsions, stereotyped perceptions, expectations of doom, or inordinate despair." For the "slum dweller," freedom was limited by poverty, unemployment, and segregation. Like mental illness, poverty and discrimination led to the "restriction of opportunity and a narrowness of choice." Both social action and psychotherapy, he argued, were designed to increase the range of options available to individuals—"in short, to enhance freedom." A slave owner, he argued somewhat philosophically, was no more free than his slaves, since "the range of his behavior is limited by his role as the owner of men." Calling for social solidarity, Dumont argued that the "communality" of the human experience led victims to "share the common burden of guilt with the criminal."[112] A shared aspiration for social freedom, Dumont summarized, was an aspiration for mental health.

Yet alongside this view of social commonality and the parallel he drew between mental health and freedom, Dumont's writing was rife with medical metaphors. The riots were an "iatrogenic disease"; in inner cities, it was necessary to "drain an abscess" to resolve urban violence. Nevertheless, the solutions Dumont suggested were clearly political.[113] Treating "this ailing organism," he argued, required a "redistribution of the wealth and resources of this country on a scale that has never been imagined."[114] His usage of medical terminology and the basis of sensory deprivation theory lent "scientific" validity to an extremely radical social proposal.

The Final Report

The Kerner Commission's final report contains accounts of the different forms of deprivation that were evident throughout the commission's deliberations and in the testimonies it heard. The document is riddled with inconsistencies. The introduction, a powerful indictment of white racism, argues that the nation was "moving toward two societies, one black, one white—separate and unequal." "White society," the report forcefully maintained, was "deeply implicated in the ghetto." Yet this introduction, written by Lindsay, the commission's most liberal member, was prepared separately from the rest of the report and did not reflect the commission's main conclusions. Circulated before the full report was released, these sentences became closely identified with the report, although they were largely divorced from the report's other conclusions, which made scarce reference to white racism.[115] In fact, other commission members later recalled that Lindsay threatened to withhold his signature from the report if the stark statements in his introduction were rephrased.[116]

In contrast to the tone set in the introduction, other chapters readily adopted the discourse of cultural deprivation and the emphasis on the pathology of the black family.[117] The main argument was the long-standing deprivation of the African American community and the need for compensation or "enrichment" to avoid further rioting. Yet the interpretations of the different forms of deprivation varied among the chapters.

Relative deprivation was one of the main frameworks through which the report interpreted the causes of the riots, reflecting much of the expert testimony it had evaluated. Lindsay's introduction argued that pervasive discrimination and segregation in employment, education, and housing excluded African Americans "from the benefits of economic progress." While "most whites and some Negroes outside the ghetto have prospered to a degree unparalleled in the history of civilization," the media "flaunted" this affluence to poor and unemployed urban African Americans, contributing to the "explosive mixture" that led to riots.[118] Similar themes appeared throughout the report: The ill effects of poverty and discrimination combined with a growing gap with white affluent society to create feelings of frustration and deprivation.[119] Accordingly, the report recommended not only encouraging integration but specifically providing "ghetto enrichment."[120] This enrichment would be "designed to offset the effects of Negro segregation and deprivation in large city ghettoes." Increased federal spending on education, housing, employment, job training, and social services was needed to counter deprivation and segregation.[121] Compensating for deprivation thus provided the scaffolding on which all of the report's findings and recommendations were hung.

Other forms of deprivation that figured in the report implicated the structure of African American society and family life rather than the structure of a racist American society. In chapter 7, "Unemployment, Family Structure, and Social Disorganization," the Kerner Commission reiterated the standard themes of the destructive psychological effects of unemployment and underemployment on black men who could not fulfill their roles as family providers and the detrimental effects of large-scale female employment. The report was highly critical of female-headed fatherless families. The ill effects of fatherlessness were further exacerbated when women were forced to work outside of the home, leaving children to roam the streets. Thus, the "image of success" for these children was the "street hustler."[122] This description echoed the Moynihan Report in highlighting the "handicap" of "poverty and deprivation" that led to a "culture of poverty." This chapter emphasized the interrelations among economic, parental, and cultural deprivation and their causal role in creating the conditions leading to urban riots.

The Kerner Report's "Recommendations for National Action" addressed employment, education, the welfare system, and housing. The educational recommendations demonstrated that the Kerner Commission had internalized the prevailing educational discourse on the necessity of compensatory education to combat cultural deprivation. Emphasizing the "debilitating effect" of a "disadvantaged environment" on learning ability and highlighting the "language deprivation" and "conceptual disabilities" of children from lower-class minority homes, the report called for an increase in compensatory education programs.[123] The report recommended expanding Head Start and other preschool programs to reach more and younger children. Additional programs were proposed to target older children and teens. The "products of ghetto schools," young graduates living in low-income areas, could be targeted by a year-round program designed to improve their verbal skills.[124] Sensory deprivation was seen as part and parcel of poverty; interventions were specifically designed to provide the environmental stimulation supposedly lacking in the homes of low-income families.

Yet the usage of the framework of deprivation transcended the commonly invoked tropes of maternal, sensory, and cultural deprivation. The report argued against racial segregation in public schools. In segregated classrooms, "disadvantaged children" were "deprived of one of the more significant ingredients of quality education: exposure to other children with strong education backgrounds."[125] The report thus relied on deprivation discourse to make an unusual argument against school segregation. African American children were commonly portrayed as deprived as a result of their disadvantaged backgrounds; in this case, deprivation was depicted as the result of the segregation itself. The Kerner Commission broadly interpreted the framework of deprivation beyond uses common at the time.

While the report itself was widely read and cited and had a significant impact on public opinion, the Johnson administration effectively buried its recommendations. Released at a time when public support for the president had reached unprecedented lows and the War on Poverty was widely criticized, the recommendations for far-reaching changes at estimated costs of up to five billion dollars were silently ignored. Johnson even refused to send thank-you notes to the members of the commission, indicating his displeasure with their report.[126]

The report was too radical for conservatives and too conservative for those who wished to see a radical restructuring of American race relations, leaving many unhappy with its conclusions and recommendations.[127] The alleviation of perceived deprivation among low-income children through programs such as Head Start garnered bipartisan support. In contrast, addressing the long-standing deprivation of African Americans was seen as politically radical and fiscally impossible. Viewing the race riots as "deprivation riots," while based on the same theories that had been used to promote and popularize early childhood intervention, shifted the burden of responsibility from "incompetent" mothers or unstimulating home environments to American society as a whole. Addressing the deprivations described throughout the report would have entailed profound structural changes that American politicians were unwilling and unable to make.

Conclusion

The rise of environmental psychology relied heavily on sensory deprivation experiments, as a wide range of often mundane phenomena, from the window view to the urge for home decoration, were interpreted by scientists from diverse backgrounds through a deprivation-oriented framework. The increasing emphasis on the relevance of urban conditions to individual psychology led both researchers and government officials to turn to analyzing the detrimental psychological effects of crowding, an endeavor that acquired new urgency after the outbreak of the race riots. Theories of deprivation shaped the Kerner Commission's interpretation of the race riots, and a framework of deprivation and compensation was omnipresent in the debate over the causes of and methods of preventing such violent outbreaks. Deprivation became a leading theory of racial violence; researchers cited forms of deprivation ranging from the sociological theory of relative deprivation to the laboratory-based theory of sensory deprivation. One urban planner explained the increase in car thefts in inner cities by arguing, apparently in complete seriousness, that "the poor feel deprived of 'automobile gratification.'"[128] Yet theories of deprivation were not used to depoliticize the riots or to portray them as the biological, essentialist outcome of a sensorily depriving environment. Proponents of deprivation theory, from Martin Luther King Jr. to psychologists testifying before the Kerner Commission, had concrete ideas regarding compensatory measures ranging from family-strengthening programs to payments for slave labor that the government should institute to address long-standing deprivations. Deprivation and compensation formed the theoretical basis of the interpretations of the causes of the urban riots and the different proposals for their prevention. This emphasis on the environment's role in creating the conditions that led to the riots relied on the newly established field of environmental psychology, which derived much of its insights and scientific legitimacy from theories of sensory deprivation. But using deprivation was not enough to ensure acceptance. Although this framework enabled politicians to rely on mental health theory to argue for otherwise controversial funding priorities, this approach went only so far. At a certain point, the content of the recommendations (an extensive reform and ultimately a redistribution of wealth through tax-funded interventions) became more important than their structure, which was based on a framework of deprivation and compensation. Relying on theories of individual psychology to argue that African American mothers or the interiors of low-income homes were depriving for young children was acceptable to both politicians and the American public at large, yet when the same theories of mental health were used to argue that American society was responsible for depriving African American adults and to suggest large-scale compensation programs, many politicians drew the line. Still, the Kerner Commission's deliberations offer a powerful example of how mental health theory could be used to call attention to pressing political problems rather than solely as a tool for medicalization and depoliticization.

Conclusion

DURING THE 2012 REPUBLICAN PRESIDENTIAL PRIMARIES, former Speaker of the House Newt Gingrich argued that children from low-income families lacked role models to teach them the importance of a good work ethic; they thus failed to understand the concept of "showing up on Monday and staying all day." They should be employed, he suggested, in jobs such as "assistant janitor" at their schools to help them learn the value of work as well as earn wages.[1] With this controversial statement, Gingrich illustrated the extent to which images of deprivation in the home lives of low-income children remain a part of current political debates. By championing middle-class and wealthy mothers who choose to stay home to raise their children while simultaneously calling for eligibility criteria that require low-income mothers of young toddlers to work to receive public assistance, conservative politicians reveal deeply ingrained views of maternal deprivation and norma-tive mothering. Time and again, politicians have enlisted a variety of images, words, and metaphors to argue that the poor have less. The interventions de-veloped to provide the poor with what they are assumed to lack, however, do not provide them with the material goods they so desperately need: income, affordable housing, or access to health care, much less such basic amenities as food and clothing. Rather, many of these interventions attempt to rem-edy perceived psychological or experiential gaps. Even Gingrich's proposal to employ poor children to clean school bathrooms was framed as a way of providing them with the experiences they sorely needed, helping them to develop a work ethic that more advantaged children would have derived from role models in their own communities.

While the poor undeniably have less of certain resources, the interven-tions examined in this volume rarely targeted these material aspects of pov-erty. From encouraging mothers to "take interest" in their children to slowly familiarizing children with different shapes and sizes, many of the 1960s War on Poverty interventions were designed to provide the poor with things they in fact did not lack or did not need. Liberal-minded experts and politicians expressed confidence that they could effectively identify and provide what the poor needed. These perceived missing components often reflected a moralizing psychological interpretation of the personal failings believed to be common among low-income and particularly minority groups. Children were unloved or unstimulated; mothers were deficient both in their homemaking abilities and in their capacity to understand and care for their children; fathers lacked self-esteem and positive masculine role models. Many of the programs examined in *What's Wrong with the Poor?* certainly had profound positive impacts on the lives of low-income families and their community, providing much-needed educational and health services. At the same time, the delivery of these services reflected deeply rooted stereotypes of what was "wrong" with society's marginalized groups.

Writing this history of the intersection of psychiatry, civil rights, and public policy in the 1960s places me in the uncomfortable position of criticizing programs I support and even admire, among them Project Head Start and the ill-fated radical community action program Mobilization for Youth. While their negative views of low-income persons of color seem abrasive to the modern reader, these experts were not racial conservatives or bigots. Their liberal politics and idealistic goal of attaining social equality through early intervention reflected the giddy optimism of the era. From Carl Bereiter, who compared African American children to deaf children who "have no language," through Bettye Caldwell, who lamented the lack of a "literacy test" for parenthood, to Susan Gray, who worried about how frying pans in disarray would interfere with children's intellectual development, the child development experts who sought to prevent and treat deprivation were deeply committed to the children they hoped to help. Rejecting hereditarian explanations for the achievement gap, these experts firmly believed that compensatory education was the key to racial equality. Similarly, members of the Kerner Commission genuinely wanted to understand the causes of civil unrest; their recommendations would have radically transformed the structure of American society. Although much of their analysis was based on deprivation theory, their attempt to make sense of urban violence was ultimately far more sympathetic to the plight of low-income inner-city African Americans than any previous interpretation.

Examining how key political moments in the 1960s embodied racially and socioeconomically biased interpretations of deprivation theory runs the risk of being read as a personal indictment of the main actors involved. That is certainly not my intention. Rather than examining how well-intentioned mental health experts could unwittingly embrace approaches that pathologized African American home life and devalued minority culture, this analysis studies the interchange between psychiatry and politics. It considers how theories of mental health were based on a collection of inherently racist and classist presuppositions. Experts privileged the white middle-class home as the normal or healthy environment; deviations from this monolithic standard were labeled pathological.

Having volunteered as a physician at the Israeli Physicians for Human Rights clinic in Jaffa, which provides health care for asylum seekers, undocumented immigrants, and Palestinians who are not Israeli citizens, I can certainly identify with experts' attempts to help the less fortunate. Dispensing advice, prescribing medication, and trying to create a safe space for these marginalized individuals, I have inevitably provided the poor with things they did not need and have been unable to offer a structural solution for the greater challenges they faced. From renewing psychiatrists' prescriptions for Ritalin while wondering whether this was the best possible response to refugee children's difficulties, to sending patients for tests to diagnose illnesses that they could not afford to treat, I have agonized over the inadequacy of our medical response in light of the structural obstacles these men and women face. While sympathetic to the attempts of the liberal-minded mental health experts, I believe that important lessons can be learned by examining their errors alongside the structural variables that predestined their interventions to remain at best problematic and at worst counterproductive.

So what went wrong with well-intentioned child development and mental health experts' valiant efforts to help the poor? Politicians proved eager to capitalize on current trends in child development, hastily assembling Project Head Start as a large-scale summer intervention despite inadequate data and planning.[2] Child development experts, aware that these programs were woefully underfunded and underresearched, cooperated in spite of their reservations, recognizing the importance of early childhood education. Academic prestige was also at stake. Apart from experts' desire to make a difference for the disadvantaged, cooperating with federal agencies had professional advantages. The significance of academic research was gauged by its ability to inform public policy. Thus, psychologist and sensory deprivation pioneer Donald Hebb was awarded the 1979 Distinguished Scientific Contributions to Child Development Award by the Society for Research in Child Devel-

opment. Hebb received the award alongside Julius Richmond and Harry
Harlow, known for his studies on monkeys raised without their mothers.[3]
Neither Hebb nor Harlow had worked with children; Richmond had directed
Project Head Start.

Politicians also influenced researchers' career trajectories through their
direct engagement with discussions of deprivation among the poor. From
President John F. Kennedy's endorsement of the theory that a lack of stimulation caused intellectual disability through Lady Bird Johnson's tour of Martin
Deutsch's IDS to the Kerner Commission's depiction of inner-city homes as
deadening and impoverished, these public figures played a powerful role in
facilitating the acceptance of theories and interventions that were aligned
with their political goals.

The ease with which researchers from loosely related fields borrowed concepts in deprivation research proved to be an additional weakness of these
interventions. Policymakers and educators regarded animal studies as directly and unproblematically applicable to humans, appropriating a vocabulary with little critical reflection. The science of toy arrangement was derived
directly from sensory deprivation experiments in a controlled laboratory setting, and maternal, nutritional, and cultural deprivation were often used interchangeably. To use literary theorist Mieke Bal's term, deprivation served as
a traveling concept that bounced among different disciplines, acquiring new
meanings and spheres of influence along the way.[4] The concept's subtlety,
specificity, and variety of meanings were often lost in policy recommendations. Policymakers eager to advance their agendas paid little heed to the
lack of data on how cultural deprivation could be targeted effectively, much
less on its actual existence. Until the late 1960s, few researchers adequately
addressed the differences or even the similarities among sensory, maternal,
and cultural deprivation.

Nevertheless, this casual conflation of concepts would likely have been
less significant had it not been complicated by the association of deprivation with poverty and race. Deprivation was not originally associated with
low-income urban blacks. Yet by the early 1960s, it had begun to provide a
language and a framework for white experts to describe a variety of traits attributed to poor blacks. In the era of civil rights and racial liberalism, experts
saw African Americans as having less rather than being less. Deprivation thus
became an ostensibly color-blind means of transforming racial inferiority into
racial disadvantage. Today, "low-income" and "inner-city" have supplanted
the no-longer-fashionable "culturally deprived"; "single-parent" families have

replaced the matriarchal families of the 1960s. All too often, these terms serve as fillers for race. Not talking about race enables us to ignore the ways in which these theories of mental health are deeply embedded in racialized presuppositions. Articulating the overlap among "cultural deprivation," "mild mental retardation," and race might have enabled well-intentioned mental health professionals to recognize their overdiagnosis of African American children as mildly intellectually disabled. It remains impossible to know whether recognizing the homogenous racial makeup of the children the Institute for Developmental Studies (IDS) served would have altered their curricular recommendations. Still, the liberal activists in the racially conscious Mississippi Head Start programs printed books that featured the lively stories of black children in their own words, explicitly celebrating the children's cultural heritage. The members of the IDS staff, in contrast, were discouraged from employing highly imaginative stories that might overwhelm their sensorily deprived charges.[5] Ignoring race thus enabled experts to discount their racial assumptions and to disregard the structural biases of the system within which they worked.

Deprivation theory allowed experts to ignore the racial overtones of their perceptions of normative behavior, maintaining a seemingly coherent theory despite obvious contradictions. Black single mothers could simultaneously be regarded as so involved in their children's lives that they were termed "matriarchs" yet at the same time be seen as causing maternal deprivation; the spoken language of African American children was compared to that of deaf children. Revealing what today seem to be unquestionably racist views, experts repeatedly argued that in many low-income African American homes, communication was "nonverbal," devoid of meaning, and often discouraged. Discounting the actual experiences of African American families, experts advanced a limited view of a healthy home environment, designing interventions to provide low-income African American children with an experience as similar as possible to that of an idealized middle-class white upbringing.

The attempts by child development experts to solve America's problems through enrichment programs for toddlers reflects what historian of education David Labaree has criticized as the trend toward "educationalizing" social problems. Using minimally effective pedagogical tools to address such pressing social problems such as racial and social inequality, Labaree argues, is a political strategy that allows those in power to avoid structural reform. Educationalizing social problems serves as a proxy for the changes American society is unwilling to make; educational opportunity becomes a poor substitute for authentic social opportunity. By projecting liberal democratic goals onto the educational system, politicians can rest assured that these goals will be implemented only within a limited scope and will not threaten the integrity of the existing social structure.[6]

Mental health and child development experts' views on early childhood intervention also reflect what has been termed the "medicalization" of education. Historians have documented the extent to which the cultivation of a healthy personality became the focus of Progressive Era education.[7] These studies have shown how the classroom came to lie within the purview of mental hygienists and later child development experts. In the process, educators embraced psychotherapeutic values and oversaw the administration of health interventions such as vaccinations and medical screening tests. *What's Wrong with the Poor?* points to a different form of medicalization: Educational programs came to represent a form of medical therapy in and of themselves. Educational enrichment programs, later subsumed under the umbrella of Project Head Start, were seen by mental health experts, politicians, and the American public as both a public health measure and a solution to America's pressing problems of racial and social inequality. Designed to overcome "environmental deficiencies," early intervention was conceptualized in medical terms that dictated day-to-day activities from playing in a sandbox to the color of each toy. Similarly, the diagnosis of poor African American children as intellectually disabled entailed placing them in "special education" classes as well as the therapeutic provision of stimulation seen to be lacking in their homes. Using this ostensibly color-blind medicalized diagnosis as a form of educational intervention enabled experts and politicians to turn educational opportunities into a sadly ineffective proxy for racial justice.

How can mental health professionals help the poor without pathologizing them? Doing so has an inherent risk of "poverty knowledge," which, as Alice O'Connor has shown, shifted the focus from economic and structural causes of poverty to the individual qualities of poor men, women, and children.[8] Social intervention, from early education to the very structure of the welfare system, has been conceptualized as a form of medical intervention, designed to fix what is wrong with low-income Americans. Since the 1960s, welfare discourse has conceptualized poverty as an illness, medicalizing social barriers to achieving ideals of individual responsibility and diligence.[9] Rather than treating the social causes of poverty and injustice, the emphasis too easily shifts to the identification and treatment of psychiatric disorders seen to afflict the poor. Present-day concerns over an apparent epidemic of depression among America's poor raises similar concerns; an approach that emphasizes individual shortcomings and their medical treatment has the potential to forestall discussions of fundamental economic change. Recommendations for social action are often couched in medical terms and presented as public health interventions.[10] Mental health experts are not trained to engage in a discussion of wider social ills; their goals should necessarily be the benefit of their individual patients. Still, they should avoid labels that medicalize poverty or locate its cause in individual defects. I do not advocate withholding treatment from low-income individuals who suffer from depression. Nevertheless, conceptualizing depression and its attendant symptoms of apathy and lack of motivation as the cause of poverty is simply a continuation of the deprivation discourse by other means. Mental health interventions serving low-income and minority populations would be well advised to focus on empowering rather than fixing individuals, drawing on their strengths, abilities, and coping mechanisms rather than correcting their deficiencies.

Clearly, this process is easier said than done, and this book is a historical analysis rather than a blueprint for change. Nevertheless, examining how mental health professionals unwittingly developed racially and socioeconomically stratified interpretations of deprivation presents a cautionary tale about the risks of using seemingly neutral theories of child development and mental health in attempts to address social problems. This approach reveals some of the hazards involved in uncritical exchanges between psychiatry and public policy. As mental health research informed public policy and public policy in turn dictated federal funding to support similar research, researchers and politicians colluded to perpetuate a certain kind of research that provided the scientific scaffolding for their policymaking. Government funding for research on "cultural deprivation" and "mild mental retardation," concepts whose utility withered within a decade and a half, could perhaps have been put to a different use.

Thus, while the poor clearly do have less, this book is a study of how mental health experts and politicians developed and propounded a theory of what they believed the poor lacked and how these deficiencies could be rectified. Only by recognizing the structural ways in which mental health discourse perpetuates and reifies negative images of low-income and minority Americans will mental health professionals be able to join forces with policymakers to make sure that the poor get what they need, not just what others think they should have.

Notes

ABBREVIATIONS

G&LBM Papers Gardner and Lois B. Murphy Papers, Archives of the History
of American Psychology, Center for the History of Psychology,
University of Akron, Akron, Ohio

JBR Julius B. Richmond

JBR Papers Julius B. Richmond Papers, 1941–2004, Modern Manuscripts
Collection, History of Medicine Division, National Library of
Medicine, Bethesda, Md., MS C 383

JMH Joseph McVicker Hunt

JMH Papers Joseph McVicker Hunt Papers, University of Illinois at
Urbana-Champaign

KC Records August Meier and John H. Bracey Jr., eds., "Part 5—Records of
the National Advisory Commission on Civil Disorder (Kerner
Commission)," in *Black Studies Research Sources: Microfilms from
Major Archival and Manuscript Collections, Civil Rights under the
Johnson Administration, 1963–1969* (Frederick, Md.: University
Publications of America, 1984–87)

MA Mary Ainsworth

MA Papers Mary Ainsworth Papers, Archives of the History of American
Psychology, Center for the History of Psychology, University
of Akron, Akron, Ohio

RAS Papers René A. Spitz Papers, Archives of the History of American
Psychology, Center for the History of Psychology, University
of Akron, Akron, Ohio

INTRODUCTION

1. Maris A. Vinovskis, *The Birth of Head Start: Preschool Education Policies in the Kennedy and Johnson Administrations* (Chicago: University of Chicago Press, 2005), 88; Edward Zigler and Sally Styfco, *The Hidden History of Head Start* (New York: Oxford University Press, 2010), 35.

2. Donald Hebb, "Donald O. Hebb," in *A History of Psychology in Autobiography*, ed. Gardner Lindzey (San Francisco: Freeman, 1980), 7:273–303; Donald Hebb, *Essay*

on Mind (Hillsdale, N.J.: Erlbaum, 1980), 90–91; Peter M. Milner and Brenda Milner, "Donald Olding Hebb, 22 July 1904–20 August 1985," *Biographical Memoirs of Fellows of the Royal Society* 42 (November 1, 1996): 192–204; Richard E. Brown and Peter M. Milner, "The Legacy of Donald O. Hebb: More Than the Hebb Synapse," *Nature Reviews Neuroscience* 4, no. 12 (2003): 1013–19.

3. Duane M. Rumbaugh, "Austin H. Riesen (1913–1996): Obituary," *American Psychologist* 53, no. 1 (1998): 60–61.

4. Donald O. Hebb, *The Organization of Behavior: A Neuropsychological Theory* (New York: Wiley, 1949).

5. Alfred McCoy, *A Question of Torture: CIA Interrogation, from the Cold War to the War on Terror* (New York: Metropolitan, 2006), 31–38; Richard E. Brown, "Alfred McCoy, Hebb, the CIA, and Torture," *Journal of the History of the Behavioral Sciences* 43, no. 2 (2007): 205–13; Alfred McCoy, "Science in Dachau's Shadow: Hebb, Beecher, and the Development of CIA Psychological Torture and Modern Medical Ethics," *Journal of the History of the Behavioral Sciences* 43, no. 4 (2007): 401–17; Naomi Klein, *The Shock Doctrine: The Rise of Disaster Capitalism* (New York: Metropolitan/Holt, 2007), 33–41.

6. McCoy, "Science in Dachau's Shadow," 404.

7. Donald O. Hebb, introduction to *Sensory Deprivation: A Symposium Held at Harvard Medical School*, ed. Philip Solomon, Philip E. Kubzansky, P. Herbert Leiderman Jr., Jack H. Mendelson, Richard Trumbull, and Donald Wexler (Cambridge: Harvard University Press, 1961), 6–7.

8. McCoy, *Question of Torture*, 31–38; Brown, "Alfred McCoy," 205–7.

9. Donald O. Hebb, Woodburn Heron, and W. H. Bexton, "The Effect of Isolation upon Attitude, Motivation, and Thought," in *Fourth Symposium, Military Medicine I* (Ottawa, Ont.: Defense Research Board, 1952).

10. Brown, "Alfred McCoy," 207; McCoy, "Science in Dachau's Shadow," 405.

11. W. H. Bexton, Woodburn Heron, and T. H. Scott: "Effects of Decreased Variation in the Sensory Environment," *Canadian Journal of Psychology* 8, no. 2 (1954): 70–76.

12. Mark Shainblum, "The King of (Understanding) Pain: Q&A with Ronald Melzack," *McGill University Headway* 4, no. 1 (2009): 23–25.

13. McCoy, *Question of Torture*, 38, 40.

14. The 1958 conference proceedings were published as Solomon et al., *Sensory Deprivation*.

15. Ronald Melzack and William R. Thompson, "Effects of Early Experience on Social Behaviour," *Canadian Journal of Psychology* 10, no. 2 (1956): 82–90; Eugene F. Gauron and Wesley C. Becker, "The Effects of Early Sensory Deprivation on Adult Rat Behavior under Competition Stress," *Journal of Comparative and Physiological Psychology* 52, no. 6 (1959): 689–93; James M. Sprague, William W. Chambers, and Eliot Stellar, "Attentive, Affective, and Adaptive Behavior in the Cat: Sensory Deprivation of the Forebrain by Lesions in the Brain Stem Results in Striking Behavioral Abnormalities," *Science* 133, no. 3447 (1961): 165–73; Stephen S. Fox, "Self-Maintained Sensory Input and Sensory Deprivation in Monkeys," *Journal of Comparative and Physiological Psychology* 55, no. 4 (1962): 438–44; Richard Held and Alan Hein, "Movement-Produced Stimulation in the Development of Visually Guided Behavior," *Journal of Comparative and Physiological Psychology* 56, no. 5 (1963): 872–76; Torsten N. Wiesel and David H.

Hubel, "Effects of Visual Deprivation on Morphology and Physiology of Cells in the Cat's Lateral Geniculate Body," *Journal of Neurophysiology* 26, no. 6 (1963): 978–93; Joseph McVicker Hunt, "Psychological Development: Early Experience," *Annual Review of Psychology* 30, no. 1 (1979): 129–34.

16. Philip Solomon, Jack Mendelson, Herbert Leiderman, and Donald Wexler, "Sensory Deprivation: A Review," *American Journal of Psychiatry* 114, no. 4 (1957): 357; Solomon et al., *Sensory Deprivation*, 1; Stuart C. Miller, "Ego-Autonomy in Sensory Deprivation, Isolation, and Stress," *International Journal of Psycho-Analysis* 43 (January–February 1962): 1–20.

17. Eugene Ziskind, Harold Jones, William Filante, and Jack Goldberg, "Observations on Mental Symptoms in Eye Patched Patients: Hypnagogic Symptoms in Sensory Deprivation," *American Journal of Psychiatry* 116, no. 10 (1960): 893–900; William Filante, Jack Goldberg, Harold Jones, and Eugene Ziskind, "Sensory Deprivation on an Eye Service—Its Significance and Management," *California Medicine* 96, no. 3 (1960): 355–56; Reginald Lourie, interview, May 10, 1977, 8, Milton J. E. Senn, American Child Guidance Clinic and Child Psychiatry Movement Interview Collection, 1975–1978, Modern Manuscripts Collection, History of Medicine Division, National Library of Medicine, Bethesda, Md., OH 76.

18. C. Wesley Jackson, John Pollard, and E. W. Kansky, "The Application of Findings from Experimental Sensory Deprivation to Cases of Clinical Sensory Deprivation," *American Journal of Medical Science* 243 (May 1962): 558–63.

19. Karl Menninger, *Theory of Psychoanalytic Technique* (New York: Basic Books, 1958), 52–53; David Rapaport, "The Theory of Ego Autonomy: A Generalization," *Bulletin of the Menninger Clinic* 22, no. 1 (1958): 62; Miller, "Ego-Autonomy," 6.

20. "Tank Test Linked to Brainwashing: U.S. and Canadian Scientists Report to Congress on Their Experiments," *New York Times*, April 15, 1956; William R. Thompson and Ronald Melzack, "Early Environment," *Scientific American* 194, no. 1 (1956): 38–42; Woodburn Heron, "The Pathology of Boredom," *Scientific American* 196, no. 1 (1957): 52–56; John A. Osmundsen, "Psychosis Linked to Heart Surgery: Many Patients Subject to Post-Operative Delusions," *New York Times*, August 6, 1965; Norman Rosenzweig, "Sensory Deprivation and Schizophrenia: Some Clinical and Theoretical Similarities," *American Journal of Psychiatry* 116, no. 4 (1959): 326–29.

21. Eleanor Leacock, ed., *The Culture of Poverty: A Critique* (New York: Simon and Schuster, 1971), based on papers from the 1966 American Anthropological Association meeting; Stephen Baratz and Joan Baratz, "Early Childhood Intervention: The Social Science Base of Institutional Racism," *Harvard Educational Review* 40, no. 1 (1970): 29–50; William Ryan, *Blaming the Victim* (London: Orbach and Chambers, 1971), 7.

22. Edward Zigler and Jeanette Valentine, eds. *Project Head Start: A Legacy of the War on Poverty* (New York: Free Press, 1979); Vinovskis, *Birth of Head Start*; Zigler and Styfco, *Hidden History*.

CHAPTER ONE

1. John Bowlby, "Forty-Four Juvenile Thieves: Their Characters and Home-Life," *International Journal of Psychoanalysis* 25 (1944): 19–53, 107–28.

2. John Bowlby, *Maternal Care and Mental Health: A Report Prepared on Behalf of the World Health Organization as a Contribution to the United Nations Programme for the Welfare of Homeless Children* (Geneva: World Health Organization, 1951), 11–12.

3. Marga Vicedo, "The Social Nature of the Mother's Tie to her Child: John Bowlby's Theory of Attachment in Post-War America," *British Journal of the History of Science* 44, no. 3 (2011): 401–26.

4. John Bowlby, *Child Care and the Growth of Love*, abridged and ed. M. Fry (Harmondsworth: Penguin, 1953); Jeremy Holmes, *John Bowlby and Attachment Theory* (London: Routledge, 1993), 38–49; Vicedo, "Social Nature," 406.

5. Holmes, *John Bowlby*, 45–48; Rose Cleary, "Bowlby's Theory of Attachment and Loss: A Feminist Reconsideration," *Feminism and Psychology* 9, no. 1 (1999): 32–42.

6. Juliet Mitchell, *Psychoanalysis and Feminism* (New York: Pantheon, 1974), 228–29.

7. One review of Robert L. Patton and Lytt I. Gardner, *Growth Failure in Maternal Deprivation* (Springfield: Thomas, 1963), argued that "maternal deprivation has now become one of the clichés of modern pediatrics, sociology and popular journalism" ("Review of *Growth Failure in Maternal Deprivation*," *Archives of Disease in Childhood* 39, no. 204 [1964]: 208).

8. Patton and Gardner, *Growth Failure*, xi.

9. Mary D. S. Ainsworth, "Mary Salter Ainsworth," in *Models of Achievement: Reflections of Eminent Women in Psychology*, ed. Agnes N. O'Connell and Nancy Felipe Russo (New York: Columbia University Press, 1983), 200–219; Mary Main, "Mary D. Salter Ainsworth: Tribute and Portrait," *Psychoanalytic Inquiry* 19, no. 5 (1999): 682–776.

10. Frank A. Pederson, "Leon J. Yarrow (1921–1982)," *American Psychologist* 40, no. 10 (1985): 1137.

11. Leon Yarrow, "Maternal Deprivation: Toward an Empirical and Conceptual Re-Evaluation," *Psychological Bulletin* 58, no. 6 (1961): 480.

12. Ibid., 486.

13. MA to John Bowlby, September 18, 1959, box M3168, folder 1, MA Papers.

14. Ibid.

15. MA to Leon Yarrow, October 12, 1963, box M3167, folder 4, MA Papers.

16. Lawrence Casler, "Maternal Deprivation: A Critical Review of the Literature," *Monographs of the Society for Research in Child Development* 26, no. 2 (1961): 14–18.

17. Ibid., 49.

18. Ibid., 22–24, 34–42.

19. MA to James Robertson, November 18, 1961, box M3167, folder 3, MA Papers.

20. MA to William E. Martin, November 14, 1961, box M3167, folder 3, MA Papers; MA to James Robertson, November 18, 1961, box M3167, folder 3, MA Papers.

21. Mary Ainsworth, "The Effects of Maternal Deprivation: A Review of Findings and Controversy in the Context of a Research Strategy," in *Deprivation of Maternal Care: A Reassessment of its Effects* (Geneva: World Health Organization, 1962), 156.

22. Peter Warren to MA, October 29, 1963, box M3168, folder 6, MA Papers.

23. MA to John Ware, May 11, 1973, box M3167, folder 7, MA Papers.

24. Mitchell Neiman to MA, January 22, 1962, box M 3169, folder 1, MA Papers. A former colleague of Zubek, Lois Brockman, described Ainsworth and Zubek's collegial relations (interview by author, August 27, 2009, Winnipeg, Manitoba).

25. MA to Allen Robinson, November 4, 1965, box M3169, folder 4, MA Papers.

26. MA to JMH, April 12, 1966, box M3169, folder 5, MA Papers. Still, Ainsworth retained her primarily psychoanalytic worldview. When asked about allowing mothers to touch their premature newborn babies while they were in incubators, she speculated that the major benefit would be not in the babies' reaction (whether they would be stimulated adequately) but rather in the mother's bonding to the child through the use of touch (MA to Linda Booth Rapoport, February 7, 1966, box 3169, folder 5, MA Papers).

27. MA to John Bowlby, December 1, 1968, box M3170, folder 4, MA Papers.

28. René Spitz, "Hospitalism: An Inquiry into the Genesis of Psychiatric Conditions in Early Childhood," *Psychoanalytic Study of the Child* 1 (1945): 53–74; René Spitz and Katharine Wolf, "Anaclitic Depression: An Inquiry into the Genesis of Psychiatric Conditions in Early Childhood," *Psychoanalytic Study of the Child* 2 (1946): 313–42.

29. Conference program, Leo Kanner Papers, box 100697, folder 92, Melvin Sabshin Library and Archives, American Psychiatric Association, Alexandria, Va.

30. See box M2114, folder 16, RAS Papers.

31. René Spitz, "Some Measurements and Clinical Observations of the Effects of Social Starvation in Infants," November 7, 1955, box M2114, folder 16, RAS Papers.

32. In a note to Spitz from his assistant and editor, W. Godfrey Coliner, concerning Spitz's review of Bowlby's *Grief and Mourning in Infancy*, Coliner wrote, "It seems to me that RAS [René A. Spitz] should state that in addition to locomotion and motility, the sensory deprivation should be taken into account. . . . In view of the advances in RAS thinking (in connection with Von Senden, Hebb etc) this will fit in." Although these comments were not incorporated in the final version of the review, they are indicative of Spitz's thought as perceived by one of his closest collaborators. See W. Godfrey Coliner to René A. Spitz, ca. July 1960, box M2115, folder 7, RAS Papers.

33. René Spitz, "Commentary," September 9, 1964, box M2124, folder 11, RAS Papers.

34. Cited in Sidney Cohen, "Contact Deprivation in Infants," *Psychosomatics* 7, no. 2 (1966): 86, 88.

35. Ibid., 88.

36. These three studies examined the influence of different kinds of sensory stimulation on institutionalized infants in New York. These infants had been placed in group care mainly because of their families' inability to care for them; all were considered healthy. See Lawrence Casler, "Supplementary Auditory and Vestibular Stimulation: Effects on Institutionalized Infants," *Journal of Experimental Child Psychology* 19, no. 3 (1975): 456–63; Lawrence Casler, "The Effects of Extra Tactile Stimulation on a Group of Institutionalized Infants," *Genetic Psychology Monographs* 71, no. 1 (1965): 137–75; Lawrence Casler, "The Effects of Supplementary Verbal Stimulation on a Group of Institutionalized Infants," *Journal of Child Psychology and Psychiatry* 6, no. 1 (1965): 19–27.

37. Casler, "Effects of Extra Tactile Stimulation," 149.

38. Ibid., 151.

39. Ibid., 171.

40. Ibid., 170.

41. For a review of the history of day care in the United States, see Elly Singer, *Child-Care and the Psychology of Development* (New York: Routledge, 1992); Sonya

Michel, *Children's Interests/Mother's Rights* (New Haven: Yale University Press, 1999); Elizabeth Rose, *A Mother's Job: The History of Day Care, 1890–1960* (New York: Oxford University Press, 1999). For an older but still pertinent analysis, see Margaret O'Brien Steinfels, *Who's Minding the Children?: The History and Politics of Day Care in America* (New York: Simon and Schuster, 1973); Pamela Roby, ed., *Child Care—Who Cares* (New York: Basic Books, 1975).

42. Sheila M. Rothman, "Other People's Children: The Day Care Experience in America," *Public Interest* 30 (Winter 1973): 11–27; Michel, *Children's Interests*, 133–36, 175–78.

43. Julia Wrigley, "Do Young Children Need Intellectual Stimulation?: Experts' Advice to Parents, 1900–1985," *History of Education Quarterly* 29, no. 1 (1989): 41–75; Maris A. Vinovskis, "Early Childhood Education: Then and Now," *Daedalus* 122, no. 1 (1993): 160–61.

44. Michel, *Children's Interests*, 155.

45. Denise Riley, *War in the Nursery* (London: Virago, 1983), 92–108.

46. Lois Wladis Hoffman, "The Decision to Work," in *The Employed Mother in America*, ed. F. Ivan Nye and Lois Wladis Hoffman (Chicago: Rand McNally, 1963), 33; Lawrence J. Sharp and F. Ivan Nye, "Maternal Mental Health," in *Employed Mother*, ed. Nye and Hoffman, 310.

47. See, for example, Florence A. Ruderman, "Family and Personal Characteristics of Working and Nonworking Mothers," in *Child Care and Working Mothers: A Study of Arrangements Made for Daytime Care of Children* (New York: Child Welfare League of America, 1968), 163–206; Alberta E. Siegel and Miriam B. Haas, "The Working Mother: A Review of the Research," *Child Development* 34 (1963): 523–27; Hoffman, "Decision to Work."

48. Florence A. Ruderman, "Conceptualizing Needs for Day Care: Some Conclusions Drawn from the Child Welfare League Day Care Project," *Child Welfare* 44, no. 3 (1965): 208–9.

49. Bettye M. Caldwell and Julius B. Richmond, "The Children's Center in Syracuse, New York," in *Early Child Care: The New Perspectives*, ed. Caroline A. Chandler, Reginald S. Lourie, and Anne DeHuff Peters (New York: Atherton, 1968), 341.

50. Singer, *Child-Care*, 122.

51. Julius B. Richmond, "Paediatric Aspects of Day Care and Institutional Care," in *Care of Children in Day Centres*, ed. Francoise Davidson (Geneva: World Health Organization, 1963), 102–3.

52. Bettye M. Caldwell and Julius B. Richmond, "Programmed Day Care for the Very Young Child: A Preliminary Report," *Journal of Marriage and Family* 26, no. 4 (1964): 486.

53. Ibid., 487–88.

54. Caldwell and Richmond, "Children's Center," 346.

55. Bettye M. Caldwell, Charlene Wright, Alice Honig, and Jordan Tannenbaum, "Infant Day Care and Attachment," *American Journal of Orthopsychiatry* 40, no. 3 (1970): 410.

56. Bettye M. Caldwell, "What Is the Optimal Learning Environment for the Young Child?," *American Journal of Orthopsychiatry* 37, no. 1 (1967): 10, 15, 18.

57. Milton Willner, "Day Care: A Reassessment," *Child Welfare* 44, no. 3 (1965): 130.

58. John E. Hansan and Kathryn Pemberton, "Day Care: A Therapeutic Milieu," *Child Welfare* 44, no. 3 (1965): 150, 153–54.

59. Phillip J. Obermiller, "Cincinnati's 'Second Minority': The Emergence of Appalachian Advocacy, 1953–1973," *Appalachian Journal* 24, no. 3 (1997): 274–95.

60. Eleanor Hosley, "Culturally Deprived Children in Day-Care Programs," *Children* 10, no. 5 (1963): 176.

61. Hosley described the "children's tragic expressions on how they feel about belonging to a discriminated against minority group," as she cited a five-year-old African American child who said he would rather be a rhinoceros than be black (ibid., 179).

62. American Institute for Research in the Behavioral Sciences, *The Day Nursery Association of Cleveland, Cleveland, Ohio: A Long History of Care for Children, Involvement of Parents, and Service to the Community* (Washington, D.C.: U.S. Government Printing Office, 1970), 10.

63. Lois B. Murphy, "The Consultant in a Day Care Center for Deprived Children," *Children* 15, no. 3 (1968): 99–100.

64. Ann D. Murray, "Maternal Employment Reconsidered: Effects on Infants," *American Journal of Orthopsychiatry* 45, no. 5 (1974): 780.

65. David Weikart and Dolores Lambie, "Preschool Intervention through a Home Teaching Program," in *Disadvantaged Child*, vol. 2, *Head Start and Early Intervention*, ed. Jerome Hellmuth (New York: Brunner/Mazal, 1968), 445, 494, 495.

66. Lois B. Murphy, "The Assessment of Infants and Young Children," in *Early Child Care*, ed. Chandler, Lourie, and Peters, 111.

67. Mary Ainsworth and Silvia Bell, "Mother-Infant Interaction and the Development of Competence," in *The Growth of Competence*, ed. Kevin Connolly and Jerome Bruner (London: Academic, 1974), 116.

68. Singer, *Child Care*, 116–18; Ralph Scott, *Research and Early Childhood: The Home Start Project* (Washington, D.C.: U.S. Office of Education, 1972).

69. Greta G. Fein and Alison Clarke-Stewart, *Day Care in Context* (New York: Wiley, 1973), 189–90. Lois B. Murphy wrote that middle-class mothers are "intuitive 'Skinnerians,'" as they "spontaneously reinforce the responses initiated by the infant which fit the picture of positive development" (Day Care Guidelines 1961–1966, Appendix—February 22, 1966, box 48, folder 3, Lois B. Murphy Papers, Modern Manuscripts Collection, History of Medicine Division, National Library of Medicine, Bethesda, Md., MS C 280c).

70. Lois B. Murphy, "Assessment of Infants," 95.

71. Murphy referred directly to the "mothering" provided for deprived children at day care facilities that would compensate for the inadequacies of their home lives (Lois B. Murphy to Emma Peters, March 24, 1966, box 44, folder 1, Lois B. Murphy Papers).

72. Caldwell and Richmond, "Children's Center," 341.

73. Lyndon B. Johnson, "Statement by the President upon Signing the Social Security Amendments and upon Appointing a Commission to Study the Nation's Welfare Programs," January 2, 1968, http://www.presidency.ucsb.edu/ws/?pid=28915.

74. Iris Rotberg to author, March 27, 2010; President's Commission on Income Main-

tenance Programs, *Poverty amid Plenty: The American Paradox* (Washington, D.C.: U.S. Government Printing Office, 1969), 62–63.

75. MA to Iris Rotberg, July 1, 1968, box M3170, folder 3, MA Papers.

76. Iris Rotberg to MA, July 22, 1968, box M3170, folder 3, MA Papers.

77. President's Commission on Income Maintenance Programs, *Poverty amidst Plenty*, 74–75.

78. Ibid.

79. Marisa Chappell, *The War on Welfare: Family, Poverty, and Politics in Modern America* (Philadelphia: University of Pennsylvania Press, 2010), 60–63.

80. Jill Quadagno, *The Color of Welfare: How Racism Undermined the War on Poverty* (New York: Oxford University Press, 1994), 121–24; Chappell, *War on Welfare*, 65–105; David Courtwright, *No Right Turn: Conservative Politics in a Liberal America* (Cambridge: Harvard University Press, 2010), 80–81.

81. Alice O'Connor, "The False Dawn of Poor-Law Reform: Nixon, Carter, and the Quest for a Guaranteed Income," in *Loss of Confidence: Politics and Policy in the 1970s*, ed. David Robertson (University Park: Pennsylvania State University Press, 1998), 99–129; Martha Derthick, *Policymaking for Social Security* (Washington, D.C.: Brookings Institution Press, 1979), 167–72.

82. Ron Hasking, *Work over Welfare: The Inside Story of the 1996 Welfare Reform Law* (Washington, D.C.: Brookings Institution Press, 2006), 340–45; Frank Stricker, *How America Lost the War on Poverty—And How to Win It* (Chapel Hill: University of North Carolina Press, 2007), 210–31; Kenneth Neubeck and Noel A. Cazenave, *Welfare Racism: Playing the Race Card against America's Poor* (New York: Routledge, 2001), 145–76.

83. Richard Nixon, "Veto of the Economic Opportunity Amendments of 1971 December 9, 1971," http://www.presidency.ucsb.edu/ws/?pid=3251.

84. Christopher Howard, *The Hidden Welfare State: Expenditures and Social Policy in the United States* (Princeton: Princeton University Press, 1997).

85. Michel, *Children's Interests*, 281–90.

86. Ibid., 1.

87. David Rothman, *Beginnings Count: The Technological Imperative in American Health Care* (New York: Oxford University Press, 1997), 3–14.

88. Ibid., 87–110.

89. William Roth, "The Politics of Daycare," *Society* 19, no. 2 (1982): 64–68; Kimberly Morgan, "A Child of the Sixties: The Great Society, the New Right, and the Politics of Federal Child Care," *Journal of Policy History* 13, no. 2 (2001): 223–43; Edward Zigler and Sally Styfco, *The Hidden History of Head Start* (New York: Oxford University Press, 2010), 162–75.

90. For a thorough analysis, see Noel A. Cazenave, "Maximum Feasible Participation Meets 'Black Power' and the White Backlash: The Struggle over Community Action in Syracuse," in *The Urban Racial State: Managing Race Relations in American Cities* (Lanham, Md.: Rowman and Littlefield, 2011), 85–102; Morgan, "Child of the Sixties," 228–32.

91. Zigler and Styfco, *Hidden History*, 172–73.

92. Morgan, "Child of the Sixties," 234; Carole Joffe, "Why the United States Has No Child-Care Policy," in *Families, Politics, and Public Policy*, ed. Irene Diamond (New

York: Longman, 1983), 172; Roth, "Politics of Daycare," 62–69. Reginald Lourie, who had testified before Congress regarding the benefits of early education, recalled that Vice President Spiro Agnew vehemently opposed the bill, arguing that "Lourie wants to Sovietize American Children" (Reginald Lourie, interview, May 10, 1977, 17, Milton J. E. Senn, American Child Guidance Clinic and Child Psychiatry Movement Interview Collection, 1975–1978, Modern Manuscripts Collection, History of Medicine Division, National Library of Medicine, Bethesda, Md., OH 76).

93. Zigler and Styfco, *Hidden History*, 167–70; Morgan, "Child of the Sixties," 224–27.

94. Cited in Dean J. Kotlowski, *Nixon's Civil Rights: Politics, Principle, and Policy* (Cambridge: Harvard University Press, 2001), 249.

95. Ibid., 247–50.

96. Ibid., 250–56.

97. Richard Nixon, "Special Message to the Congress on the Nation's Antipoverty Programs, February 19, 1969," http://www.presidency.ucsb.edu/ws/?pid=2397; Urie Bronfenbrenner and Jerome Bruner, "The President and the Children," *New York Times*, January 31, 1972.

98. Joseph Clark to Paul Gyorgy, August 8, 1968, box 27, folder 2, JBR Papers; Urie Bronfenbrenner to Carl Perkins, August 9, 1968, box 1, folder 78, Urie Bronfenbrenner Papers, 23-13-954, Division of Rare and Manuscript Collections, Cornell University Library, Ithaca, N.Y. See also Maris A. Vinovskis, *The Birth of Head Start: Preschool Education Policies in the Kennedy and Johnson Administrations* (Chicago: University of Chicago Press, 2005), 126–28.

99. Nixon, "Special Message to the Congress on the Nation's Antipoverty Programs, February 19, 1969."

100. Nixon, "Veto of the Economic Opportunity Amendments."

101. Michel, *Children's Interests*, 154; Sheila M. Rothman, "Other People's Children," 22.

CHAPTER TWO

1. Michael B. Katz, *The Undeserving Poor: From the War on Poverty to the War on Welfare* (New York: Pantheon, 1989), 16–66.

2. Oscar Lewis, *Five Families: Mexican Case Studies in the Culture of Poverty* (New York: Basic Books, 1959), 2; Katz, *Undeserving Poor*, 18–23.

3. Lewis, *Five Families*, 2.

4. Oscar Lewis, *The Children of Sánchez: Autobiography of a Mexican Family* (New York: Random House, 1961); David Price, *Threatening Anthropology: McCarthyism and the FBI's Surveillance of Activist Anthropologists* (Durham: Duke University Press, 2004), 246–48; Alden Whitman, "Oscar Lewis, Author and Anthropologist, Dead," *New York Times*, December 18, 1970.

5. Michael Harrington, *The Other America: Poverty in the United States* (New York: Macmillan, 1962); Maurice Isserman, *The Other American: The Life of Michael Harrington* (New York: Public Affairs, 2000), 215–16.

6. James T. Patterson, *Grand Expectations: The United States, 1945–1974* (New York: Oxford University Press, 1996), 532–40; James T. Patterson, *Freedom Is Not Enough: The Moynihan Report and America's Struggle over Black Family Life from LBJ to Obama* (New

York: Basic Books, 2010), 30–33; Maurice Isserman, "Michael Harrington: Warrior on Poverty," *New York Times*, June 19, 2009.

7. In fact, some observers refer to cultural deprivation theory as a derivative of the culture of poverty approach. See, for example, K. Ann Renninger and Irving E. Sigel, *Handbook of Child Psychology*, vol. 4, *Child Psychology in Practice* (Hoboken, N.J.: Wiley, 2006), 708. Others have used the terms interchangeably. See Diane Ravitch, *The Troubled Crusade: American Education, 1945–1980* (New York: Basic Books, 1983), 157; Katz, *Undeserving Poor*, 37–38. Still others bundle the terms together. See Jerald Podair, *The Strike That Changed New York: Blacks, Whites, and the Ocean-Brownsville Crisis* (New Haven: Yale University Press, 2002), 59–65.

8. Frank Riessman, *The Culturally Deprived Child* (New York: Harper and Row, 1962), 1.

9. Rodger L. Hurley, *Poverty and Mental Retardation: A Causal Relationship* (New York: Vintage, 1969), 71–72; James E. Birren and Robert D. Hess, "Influences of Biological, Psychological, and Social Deprivations upon Learning and Performance," in *Perspectives on Human Deprivation: Biological, Psychological, and Sociological* (Washington, D.C.: U.S. Department of Health, Education, and Welfare, 1968), 96.

10. Thomas Kiffmeyer, *Reformers to Radicals: The Appalachian Volunteers and the War on Poverty* (Lexington: University Press of Kentucky, 2008); Katz, *Undeserving Poor*, 23.

11. Katz, *Undeserving Poor*, 24–25; Benjamin Bloom, Allison Davis, and Robert Hess, *Compensatory Education for Cultural Deprivation* (Chicago: Holt, Rinehart, and Winston, 1965), 5; Daryl M. Scott, *Contempt and Pity: Social Policy and the Image of the Damaged Black Psyche, 1880–1996* (Chapel Hill: University of North Carolina Press, 1997), 143–44.

12. William F. Brazziel, "Two Years of Head Start," *Phi Delta Kappan*, March 1967, 348.

13. Clark's earliest critique of the cultural deprivation approach appears in Kenneth Clark, "Clash of Cultures in the Classroom," *Equity and Excellence in Education* 1, no. 4 (1963): 7–14.

14. Kenneth Clark, *Dark Ghetto: Dilemmas of Social Power* (New York: Harper and Row, 1965), 129–33.

15. Eleanor Leacock, ed., *The Culture of Poverty: A Critique* (New York: Simon and Schuster, 1971), based on papers from the 1966 American Anthropological Association meeting.

16. Charles Valentine, "The 'Culture of Poverty': Its Scientific Significance and Its Implications for Action," in *Culture of Poverty*, ed. Leacock, 218. See also Frank Stricker, *Why America Lost the War on Poverty and How to Win It* (Chapel Hill: University of North Carolina Press, 2007), 117–56; Katz, *Undeserving Poor*, 185–235.

17. S. M. Miller and Frank Riessman, *Social Class and Social Policy* (New York: Basic Books, 1968), 99.

18. Stephen Baratz and Joan Baratz, "Early Childhood Intervention: The Social Science Base of Institutional Racism," *Harvard Educational Review* 40, no. 1 (1970): 29–50.

19. William Ryan, *Blaming the Victim* (London: Orbach and Chambers, 1971), 7.

20. Richard Valencia, ed., *The Evolution of Deficit Thinking* (London: Falmer, 1997); Jeanne Ellsworth, "Inspiring Delusions: Reflections on Head Start's Enduring Popularity," in *Critical Perspectives on Project Head Start*, ed. Jeanne Ellsworth and Lynda J.

Ames (Albany: SUNY Press, 1998), 322–24; Richard Valencia, *Dismantling Contemporary Deficit Thinking: Educational Thought and Practice* (New York: Routledge, 2010).

21. Lewis, *Five Families*, 14, 16–18.

22. Lewis, *Children of Sanchez*, xxxviii.

23. President Lyndon B. Johnson, "To Fulfill These Rights," speech at Howard University, June 4, 1965, in *The Moynihan Report and the Politics of Controversy*, ed. Lee Rainwater and William Yancey (Cambridge: MIT Press, 1967); Scott, *Contempt and Pity*, 151.

24. Daniel P. Moynihan, "The Negro Family: The Case for National Action," in *Moynihan Report*, ed. Rainwater and Yancey, 5.

25. For further analyses of the Moynihan report and its reception, see Katz, *Undeserving Poor*, 24–29, 44–52; Scott, *Contempt and Pity*, 150–56; Alice O'Connor, *Poverty Knowledge: Social Science, Social Policy, and the Poor in Twentieth-Century U.S. History* (Princeton: Princeton University Press, 2001), 203–10; Ruth Feldstein, *Motherhood in Black and White* (Ithaca: Cornell University Press, 2000), 142–52.

26. Moynihan, "Negro Family," 25.

27. Ibid.

28. Moynihan quotes the studies of Thomas Pettigrew (ibid., 77–80). See Thomas Pettigrew, *A Profile of the Negro American* (Princeton: Van Nostrand, 1964), 16–17.

29. Feldstein, *Motherhood in Black and White*, 147.

30. Ibid., 166–69. For additional feminist criticism of the Moynihan report, see Leith Mullings, *On Our Own Terms: Race, Class, and Gender in the Lives of African American Women* (New York: Routledge, 1997), 116–18, 161–62.

31. Many of the early descriptions of maternal deprivation clearly referred to the lifestyles of middle-class women, as John Bowlby describes in a pamphlet dedicated to answering a question troubling many mothers at the time, "Can I leave my baby?" His answer: In some cases, leaving infants with neighbors or relatives is an "excellent" idea that will allow mothers to have "an afternoon's shopping in peace, visits to the doctor or dentist, the cinema or tea with friends" (John Bowlby, *Can I Leave My Baby?* [London: National Association for Mental Health, 1958], 6).

32. See, for example, John Bracey, August Meier, and Elliott Rudwick, eds., *Black Matriarchy: Myth or Reality?* (Belmont, Calif.: Wasworth, 1971).

33. Pettigrew, *Profile*, 15–18; Joseph White, "Toward a Black Psychology," *Ebony* 25, no. 11 (September 1970): 45.

34. Herbert Hyman and John Reed, "Black Matriarchy Reconsidered: Evidence from Secondary Analysis of Sample Surveys," *Public Opinion Quarterly* 33, no. 3 (1969): 346–54; Katheryn Dietrich, "A Reexamination of the Myth of Black Matriarchy," *Journal of Marriage and Family* 37, no. 2 (1975): 367–74; Steven Mintz and Susan Kellogg, *Domestic Revolutions: A Social History of American Family Life* (New York: Free Press, 1988), 210–12.

35. Oscar Lewis, *La Vida: A Puerto Rican Family in the Culture of Poverty* (New York: Random House, 1966), xlviii.

36. Celia Stendler-Lavatelli, "Environmental Intervention in Infancy and Early Childhood," in *Social Class, Race, and Psychological Development*, ed. Martin Deutsch, Irwin Katz, and Arthur Jensen (New York: Holt, Rinehart, and Winston, 1968), 357.

37. Kermit Wiltse, "Orthopsychiatric Programs for Socially Deprived Groups," *American Journal of Orthopsychiatry* 33, no. 5 (1963): 809.

38. Rima Apple, *Vitamania: Vitamins in American Culture* (New Brunswick, N.J.: Rutgers University Press, 1995); Kay Codell Carter, "The Germ Theory, Beriberi, and the Deficiency Theory of Disease," *Medical History* 21, no. 2 (1977): 119–36.

39. Rima Apple, "Science Gendered: Nutrition in the United States, 1840–1940," in *The Science and Culture of Nutrition, 1840–1940*, ed. Harmke Kamminga and Andrew Cunningham (Atlanta: Rodopi, 1995), 129–41; Rima Apple, "Constructing Mothers: Scientific Motherhood in the Nineteenth and Twentieth Centuries," *Social History of Medicine* 8, no. 2 (1995): 161–78.

40. Cited in Rima Apple, *Perfect Motherhood: Science and Childrearing in America* (New Brunswick, N.J.: Rutgers University Press, 2006), 117.

41. Ibid., 79–81.

42. Alan M. Kraut, *Goldberger's War: The Life and Work of a Public Health Crusader* (New York: Hill and Wang, 2003); Harry M. Marks, "Epidemiologists Explain Pellagra: Gender, Race, and Political Economy in the Work of Edgar Sydenstricker," *Journal of the History of Medicine and Allied Sciences* 58, no. 1 (2003): 34–55; Keith Wailoo, *Drawing Blood: Technology and Disease Identity in Twentieth-Century America* (Baltimore: Johns Hopkins University Press, 1997), 99–133.

43. Apple, *Vitamania*, 183.

44. Kenneth J. Carpenter, "A Short History of Nutritional Science: Part 4 (1945–1985)," *Journal of Nutrition* 133, no. 11 (2003): 3333–36.

45. Todd Tucker, *Great Starvation Experiment: Ancel Keys and the Men Who Starved for Science* (Minneapolis: University of Minnesota Press, 2007), 201–13; "Men Starve in Minnesota," *Life*, July 30, 1945, 43–46.

46. Tucker, *Great Starvation Experiment*, 206–7; Ancel Keys and Margaret Keys, *Eat Well and Stay Well* (Garden City, N.Y.: Doubleday, 1959); Ancel Keys, ed., *Coronary Heart Disease in Seven Countries* (New York: American Heart Association, 1970).

47. Tucker, *Great Starvation Experiment*, 208.

48. A. Frederick North Jr., "Health Services in Head Start," in *Project Head Start: A Legacy of the War on Poverty*, ed. Edward Zigler and Jeanette Valentine (New York: Free Press, 1979), 231–58; A. Frederick North Jr. to Gloria Bittman, May 24, 1967, box 26, folder 12, JBR Papers.

49. Alvin Schorr, "The Nonculture of Poverty," *American Journal of Orthopsychiatry* 34, no. 5 (1964): 908.

50. Ernest Austin, "Cultural Deprivation: A Few Questions," *Phi Delta Kappan* 47, no. 2 (1965): 67.

51. Daniel P. Moynihan, ed., *On Understanding Poverty* (New York: Basic Books, 1969); Alice O'Connor, *Poverty Knowledge*, 196–97.

52. Moynihan, "The Professors and the Poor," in *On Understanding Poverty*, ed. Moynihan, 21.

53. Ibid., 22.

54. Ibid., 22–26.

55. Jerome S. Bruner, "Poverty and Childhood," in *The Relevance of Education* (New York: Norton, 1971), 150.

56. Jerome S. Bruner and Kevin Connolly, "Competence: The Growth of the Person," in *The Growth of Competence*, ed. Kevin Connolly and Jerome S. Bruner (London, Academic, 1974), 310. In an oral history interview, Bruner referred to "cultural deprivation" as a "stupid idea." In the mid-1960s, Bruner recalled, he and his colleagues still endorsed an "avitaminosis" theory of cultural deprivation (Jerome S. Bruner, interview by Ronald Grele, February 18, 1999, 21–23, Columbia University Center for Oral History, New York).

57. Oscar Stine, John Saratsiotis, and Orlando Furno, "Appraising the Health of Culturally Deprived Children," *American Journal of Clinical Nutrition* 20, no. 10 (1967): 1091.

58. Sidney Werkman, Lydia Shifman, and Thomas Skelly, "Psychosocial Correlates of Iron Deficiency Anemia in Early Childhood," *Psychosomatic Medicine* 26, no. 2 (1964): 125–34.

59. For a more complete discussion, see Eduardo Duniec and Mical Raz, "Vitamins for the Soul: John Bowlby's Thesis of Maternal Deprivation, Biomedical Metaphors, and the Deficiency Model of Disease," *History of Psychiatry* 22, no. 1 (2011): 93–107.

60. President's Panel on Mental Retardation, *A Proposed Program for National Action to Combat Mental Retardation* (Washington, D.C.: U.S. Government Printing Office, 1962), 8.

61. Lois B. Murphy, "Memorandum on First Six Months of Work under Grant MH 09236-01," March 1, 1967, box M1808, folder 1, G&LBM Papers.

62. Bloom, Davis, and Hess, *Compensatory Education*, 8.

63. Ibid., 4, 22.

64. Ibid., 13–15.

65. Susan Gray and Rupert Klaus, "Brief Reflections on the Theory of Early Childhood Enrichment Programs," in *Early Education: Current Theory, Research, and Action*, ed. Robert Hess and Roberta Bear (Chicago: Aldine, 1968), 65.

66. Vera John, "The Intellectual Development of Slum Children: Some Preliminary Findings," *American Journal of Orthopsychiatry* 33, no. 5 (1963): 814–15.

67. Edward Zigler and Karen Anderson, "An Idea Whose Time Had Come: The Intellectual and Political Climate," in *Project Head Start*, ed. Zigler and Valentine, 9. Zigler was one of the few psychologists who repeatedly emphasized the problematic aspects of Head Start in the program's attitude toward poor families and their child rearing abilities. In 1975, he argued that "viewed from one perspective, HS [Head Start] may be seen as part of the problem rather than part of the solution. I am thinking here of the fact that philosophically the HS program disparages the poor. What we are in effect saying is that poor people are inadequate parents and the only salvation for their children is to put these children into the hands of HS personnel so that we might compensate for the ill-effects suffered as a result of having an inadequate family" (Edward Zigler to Stanley Thomas, July 18, 1975, box 9, folder 11, JBR Papers).

68. JMH to Lois B. Murphy, February 2, 1967, box 50, folder 1, Lois B. Murphy Papers, Modern Manuscripts Collection, History of Medicine Division, National Library of Medicine, Bethesda, Md., MS C 280c.

69. Carl Haywood, "Joseph McVicker Hunt (1906–1991)," *American Psychologist* 47, no. 8 (1992): 1050–51.

70. Joseph McVicker Hunt, "The Psychological Basis for Using Preschool Enrich-

ment as an Antidote for Cultural Deprivation," *Merrill-Palmer Quarterly* 10, no. 3 (1964): 237.

71. Ibid., 242.

72. Urie Bronfenbrenner to JMH, January 8, 1965, box 51, folder Preschool Enrichment and Cultural Deprivation, JMH Papers.

73. JMH to Urie Bronfenbrenner, January 13, 1965, box 51, folder Preschool Enrichment and Cultural Deprivation, JMH Papers.

74. Jean Sweitzer to JMH, September 29, 1964, Hunt's secretary to Sweitzer, November 2, 1964, Mrs. Thomas L. Spiegel to JMH, May 21, 1965, all in box 51, folder "Preschool Enrichment and Cultural Deprivation," JMH Papers.

75. In a letter to Julius B. Richmond, Hunt wrote of his concern of rushing into a large-scale program and without being confident of its feasibility, thus endangering the possibility of future attempts to develop more advanced programs (JMH to JBR, May 25, 1965, box 58, folder "Head Start, 1965–66," JMH Papers).

76. Basil Bernstein, "Linguistic Codes, Hesitation Phenomena, and Intelligence," *Language and Speech* 5, no. 1 (1962): 31–48; Basil Bernstein, "Social Class, Linguistic Codes, and Grammatical Elements," *Language and Speech* 5, no. 4 (1962): 221–40.

77. Basil Bernstein, "The Role of Speech in the Development and Transmission of Culture," in *Perspectives on Learning: Papers from the Bank Street Fiftieth Anniversary Invitational Symposium*, ed. Gordon Klopf and William A. Hohman (New York: Mental Health Materials Center for the Bank Street College of Education, 1967), 25.

78. Basil Bernstein, *Class, Codes, and Control: Theoretical Studies towards a Sociology of Language*, 2nd ed. (New York: Schocken, 1974), 9–10.

79. Ibid., 9.

80. Robert D. Hess and Virginia C. Shipman, "Early Experience and the Socialization of Cognitive Modes in Children," *Child Development* 36, no. 4 (1965): 870.

81. Ibid., 885.

82. For a discussion of the debate over Standard English, see Tony Bex and Richard J. Watts, *Standard English: The Widening Debate* (London: Routledge, 1999); Tony Crowley, *Standard English and the Politics of Language* (New York: Palgrave Macmillan, 2003).

83. Carl Bereiter, Siegfried Engelmann, Jean Osborn, and Philip Reidford, "An Academically Oriented Pre-School for Culturally Deprived Children," in *Pre-School Education Today*, ed. Fred Hechinger (Garden City, N.Y.: Doubleday, 1966), 112.

84. Bereiter et al., "Academically Oriented Pre-School," 113; Carl Bereiter and Siegfried Engelmann, *Teaching Disadvantaged Children in the Preschool* (Englewood Cliffs, N.J.: Prentice Hall, 1966), 30–31.

85. Bereiter et al., "Academically Oriented Pre-School," 114–15, 134; Bereiter and Engelmann, *Teaching Disadvantaged Children*, 30–31.

86. Bernstein, "Role of Speech," 15.

87. Ibid., 26.

88. Ibid., 26, 31, 34.

89. Ibid., 31–32.

90. Ibid., 33.

91. Ibid., 40.

92. Ibid., 42.

93. Ibid., 35–37.

94. Ibid., 37.

95. Ibid., 35.

96. Matthew J. Gordon, "Interview with William Labov," *Journal of English Linguistics* 34, no. 4 (2006): 343–45; William Labov, "How I Got into Linguistics and What I Got Out of It—Personal Reflections," October 1, 1997, http://www.pbs.org/speak/speech/sociolinguistics/labov/.

97. William Labov and Clarence Robins, *A Note on the Relation of Reading Failure to Peer Group Status in Urban Ghettos* (New York: Columbia University, 1967).

98. Labov delivered a paper on negative forms at a 1968 conference of the Linguistic Society of America. It was later published as William Labov, "Negative Attraction and Negative Concord in English Grammar," *Language* 48, no. 4 (1972): 773–818.

99. William Labov, "The Logic of Nonstandard English," in *The Myth of Cultural Deprivation*, ed. Nell Keddie (Harmondsworth: Penguin, 1973), 21–66.

100. Ibid., 24–25.

101. Ibid., 28–31.

102. Ibid., 33–34.

103. William Labov, "Academic Ignorance and Black Intelligence," *Atlantic Monthly* 229, no. 6 (1972): 59–67.

104. Aaron Cicourel and Hugh Mehan, "Remembering Basil Bernstein," in *A Tribute to Basil Bernstein, 1924–2000*, ed. Sally Power, Julia Brannen, Peter Aggleton, Andrew Brown, and Lynne Chisholm (London: Institute of Education Publications, 2001), 96–100; Paul Atkinson, *Language, Structure, and Reproduction: An Introduction to the Sociology of Basil Bernstein* (London: Methuen, 1985), 100–107; Ronald Wardhaugh, *An Introduction to Sociolinguistics*, 6th ed. (Malden, Mass.: Wiley-Blackwell, 2010), 360–64.

105. Labov, "Logic of Nonstandard English," 30–31.

106. Atkinson, *Language, Structure, and Reproduction*, 107–9.

107. Bernstein, *Class, Codes, and Control*, 193.

108. Ibid., 255.

109. Alan Sadovnick, "Basil Bernstein: 1924–2000," *Prospects: The Quarterly Review of Comparative Education* 31, no. 4 (2001): 690.

110. Hess and Shipman, "Early Experience," 869–86; Robert D. Hess and Virginia C. Shipman, "Early Blocks to Children's Learning," *Children* 12, no. 5 (1965): 189–94; Ellis G. Olim, Robert D. Hess, and Virginia C. Shipman, "Role of Mothers' Language Styles in Mediating Their Preschool Children's Cognitive Development," *School Review* 75, no. 4 (1967): 414–24. See also Elly Singer, *Child-Care and the Psychology of Development* (New York: Routledge, 1992), 118–20.

111. JMH to JBR, May 25, 1965, box 58, folder "Head Start 1965–66," JMH Papers. In a review article from 1975, Hunt admitted that his hypothesis that the "noise and the variety of experiences associated with the crowding of families of poverty might help to foster development in early infancy" had been proven to be "very wrong" (Joseph McVicker Hunt, "Reflections on a Decade of Early Education," *Journal of Abnormal Child Psychology* 3, no. 4 [1975]: 280).

112. Joseph McVicker Hunt, "How Children Develop Intellectually," *Children* 11, no. 3 (1964): 88–89.

113. Herbert Ginsburg, *The Myth of the Deprived Child* (Englewood Cliffs, N.J.: Prentice-Hall, 1972), 14–15.

114. Kenneth Clark, "The Cult of Cultural Deprivation," in *Children with Reading Problems*, ed. Gladys Natchez (New York: Basic Books, 1968), 180–82.

115. For a comprehensive analysis, see John P. Jackson, *Science for Segregation: Race, Law, and the Case against Brown v. Board of Education* (New York: New York University Press, 2005); Valencia, *Dismantling Contemporary Deficit Thinking*, 23–33.

116. Jackson, *Science for Segregation*, 69–92.

117. R. C. Lewontin, Steven Rose, and Leon J. Kamin, "IQ: The Rank Ordering of the World," in *The Racial Economy of Science: Toward a Democratic Future*, ed. Sandra Harding (Bloomington: Indiana University Press, 1993), 142–62.

118. For a history of intelligence testing, see Leila Zenderland, *Measuring Minds: Henry Herbert Goddard and the Origins of American Intelligence Testing* (New York: Cambridge University Press, 1997). For an approach highlighting the role of white racism, see William Wright, *Racism Matters* (Westport, Conn.: Greenwood, 1998), 133–66.

119. Barbara Beatty, "The Debate over the Young 'Disadvantaged Child': Preschool Intervention, Developmental Psychology, and Compensatory Education in the 1960s and Early 1970s," *Teachers College Record* 114, no. 6 (2012): 1–21.

120. See, for example, Frank C. J. McGurk, "The Culture Hypothesis and Psychological Tests," in *Race and Modern Science: A Collection of Essays by Biologists, Anthropologists, Sociologists, and Psychologists*, ed. Robert E. Kuttner (New York: Social Science Press, 1967), 367–81.

121. Jackson, *Science for Segregation*, 178–91. For an analysis written by a scholar who defines himself as "agnostic" regarding the biological basis of racial differences, see Raymond Wolters, *Race and Education, 1954–2007* (Columbia: University of Missouri Press, 2009), 124–54.

122. Robert L. Williams, "Black Pride, Academic Relevance, and Individual Achievement," *Counseling Psychologist* 2, no. 1 (1970): 18–22; Robert L. Williams, "A History of the Association of Black Psychologists: Early Formation and Development," *Journal of Black Psychology* 1, no. 1 (1974): 9–24; Robert L. Williams, William Dotson, Patricia Don, and Willie S. Williams, "The War against Testing: A Current Status Report," *Journal of Negro Education* 49, no. 3 (1980): 263–73.

123. Joseph McVicker Hunt, *Intelligence and Experience* (New York: Ronald, 1961); Benjamin Bloom, *Stability and Change in Human Characteristics* (New York: Wiley, 1964).

124. Hunt, *Intelligence and Experience*, 28–34; Bloom, *Stability and Change*, 77–78.

125. Sandra Condry, "History and Background of Preschool Intervention Programs and the Consortium for Longitudinal Studies," in *As the Twig Is Bent: Lasting Effects of Preschool Programs*, ed. Consortium for Longitudinal Studies (Hillsdale, N.J.: Erlbaum, 1983), 1–33; Richard Valencia and Lisa Suzuki, *Intelligence Testing and Minority Students* (Thousand Oaks, Calif.: Sage, 2001), 84–85; Sheldon White and Deborah Phillips, "Designing Head Start: Roles Played by Developmental Psychologists," in *Social Science and Policy-Making: A Search for Relevance in the Twentieth Century*, ed. David Featherman and Maris A. Vinovskis (Ann Arbor: University of Michigan Press, 2001), 96–97; Maris A. Vinovskis, *The Birth of Head Start: Preschool Education Policies*

in the Kennedy and Johnson Administrations (Chicago: University of Chicago Press, 2005), 10–11; Timothy A. Hacsi, *Children as Pawns: The Politics of Educational Reform* (Cambridge: Harvard University Press, 2002), 24–25. Education researcher David Weikart describes the importance of Hunt's book in shaping his perceptions of the environmental determinants of intelligence, recalling how he had been troubled when he realized that he could predict children's IQ solely by knowing their address (David Weikart, interview by Sharon Zane and Mary Marshall Clark, February 18, 1999, 2–70, Columbia University Center for Oral History, New York).

126. Scott, *Contempt and Pity*, 80; Alice O'Connor, *Poverty Knowledge*, 199; Thomas Pettigrew, "Negro American Intelligence: A New Look at an Old Controversy," *Journal of Negro Education* 33, no. 1 (1964): 6–25; Pettigrew, *Profile*.

127. Pettigrew, "Negro American Intelligence," 6, 8.

128. Nancy K. Innis, "Tolman and Tryon: Early Research on the Inheritance of the Ability to Learn," *American Psychologist* 47, no. 2 (1992): 190–97.

129. Pettigrew, "Negro American Intelligence," 10.

130. Ibid., 11–12.

131. Ibid., 11–12, 13.

132. MA to John Bowlby, March 23, 1965, box M3168, folder 2, MA Papers.

133. James L. Fuller, "Experiential Deprivation and Later Behavior," *Science* 158, no. 809 (1967): 1645.

134. Ibid., 1651–52.

135. Jackson, *Science for Segregation*, 60–62, 185–86; Robert Kuttner, "Why Aren't Indians 'Disadvantaged?,'" *American Mercury*, Fall 1969, 8–9.

136. Kuttner, "Why Aren't Indians 'Disadvantaged?,'" 8.

137. Kenneth Neubeck and Noel Cazenave, *Welfare Racism: Playing the Race Card against America's Poor* (New York: Routledge, 2001), 115–45.

138. Ibid., 118–35; Roger Hewitt, *White Backlash and the Politics of Multiculturalism* (New York: Cambridge University Press, 2005), 19–22.

139. Westinghouse Learning Corporation, *The Impact of Head Start* (Washington, D.C.: U.S. Department of Health Education and Welfare, 1969); Edward Zigler and Sally Styfco, *The Hidden History of Head Start* (New York: Oxford University Press, 2010), 179–84.

140. Eugene Garfield, "High Impact Science and the Case of Arthur Jensen," *Current Contents*, October 9, 1978, 652–62; Mark Snyderman and Stanley Rothman, *The IQ Controversy, the Media, and Public Policy* (New Brunswick, N.J.: Transaction, 1988), 1–4, 203–30.

141. See, for example, Frank Miele, *Intelligence, Race, and Genetics: Conversations with Arthur R. Jensen* (Boulder, Colo.: Westview, 2002), 35, 147–65; J. Philippe Rushton and Arthur Jensen, "Thirty Years of Research on Race Differences in Cognitive Ability," *Psychology, Public Policy, and Law* 11, no. 2 (2005): 280–81.

142. Jackson, *Science for Segregation*, 184–85.

143. Arthur Jensen, "The Culturally Disadvantaged and the Heredity-Environment Uncertainty," in *Disadvantaged Child*, ed. Jerome Hellmuth (Seattle: Straub and Hellmuth, 1967), 42–43.

144. Arthur Jensen, "How Much Can We Boost IQ and Scholastic Achievement?,"

in *Environment, Heredity, and Intelligence: Reprints from the Harvard Educational Review* (Cambridge: Harvard Educational Review, 1969), 60–61.

145. Ibid., 73–74.

146. Joseph McVicker Hunt, "Has Compensatory Education Failed?: Has It Been Attempted?," in *Environment, Heredity, and Intelligence*, 136–42.

147. Arthur Jensen, "Reducing the Heredity-Environment Uncertainty," in *Environment, Heredity, and Intelligence*, 230–34.

148. Frank Riessman, whose book, *The Culturally Deprived Child*, had contributed to the widespread acceptance of the theory of cultural deprivation, later changed his views to emphasize the strengths rather than the deficiencies of low-income children. In his *Social Class and Social Policy*, coauthored with Seymour Miller, he criticized theories of compensatory education and argued that the "preschool strategy was based on a loose overgeneralization of various animal experiments and special human (or inhuman) experiments on sensory deprivation" (Miller and Riessman, *Social Class and Social Policy*, 116).

149. Jerome S. Kagan, "Inadequate Evidence and Illogical Conclusions," in *Environment, Heredity, and Intelligence*, 127–28.

150. Kagan later published numerous influential works on early child development. Some results of this study appear in Jerome Kagan, *Change and Continuity in Infancy* (New York: Wiley, 1971). See also Jerome Kagan, "Jerome Kagan," in *A History of Psychology in Autobiography*, ed. Gardner Lindzey and William M. Runyan (Washington, D.C.: American Psychological Association, 2007), 9:115–53.

151. Martin Deutsch, "Happenings on the Way Back to the Forum: Social Science, IQ, and Race Differences Revisited," in *Harvard Educational Review*, Reprint Series No. 4, *Science, Heritability, and IQ* (Cambridge: Harvard Educational Review, 1969), 64–65.

152. Ibid., 84.

153. Ibid., 85.

154. William F. Brazziel, "A Letter from the South," in *Environment, Heredity, and Intelligence*, 200–208.

155. Ibid., 202, 205.

156. Ibid., 207–8.

157. Arthur Jensen, *Educability and Group Differences* (New York: Harper and Row, 1973), 277–83.

158. Ibid., 285–87.

159. William Goldfarb, "Effects of Psychological Deprivation in Infancy and Subsequent Stimulation," *American Journal of Psychiatry* 102, no. 1 (1945): 18–33.

160. William Goldfarb, interview, March 17, 1977, Milton J. E. Senn, American Child Guidance Clinic and Child Psychiatry Movement Interview Collection, 1975–1978, Modern Manuscripts Collection, History of Medicine Division, National Library of Medicine, Bethesda, Md., OH 76.

161. Scott, *Contempt and Pity*, 161–85.

162. Price, *Threatening Anthropology*, 237–54.

163. Mario Luis Small, David J. Harding, and Michèle Lamont, "Reconsidering Poverty and Culture," *Annals of the American Academy of Political and Social Science* 629 (2010): 6–27.

164. Richard Valencia and Daniel Solorzano, "Contemporary Deficit Thinking," in *Evolution of Deficit Thinking*, ed. Valencia, 160–210; Valencia, *Dismantling Contemporary Deficit Thinking*, 23–33.

CHAPTER THREE

1. Fred Powledge, *To Change a Child: A Report on the Institute for Developmental Studies* (Chicago: Anti-Defamation League, 1967), 48.

2. Daniel P. Moynihan, *Maximum Feasible Misunderstanding: Community Action in the War on Poverty* (New York: Free Press, 1969), 56; Maris A. Vinovskis, *The Birth of Head Start: Preschool Education Policies in the Kennedy and Johnson Administrations* (Chicago: University of Chicago Press, 2005), 29–30; Edward Zigler and Sally Styfco, *The Hidden History of Head Start* (New York: Oxford University Press, 2010), 6–11.

3. Susan Gray and Rupert Klaus, "An Experimental Preschool Program for Culturally Deprived Children," *Child Development* 36, no. 4 (1965): 888.

4. Susan Gray, Rupert Klaus, James Miller, and Bettye Forrester, *Before First Grade: The Early Training Project for Culturally Disadvantaged Children* (New York: Teachers College Press, 1966), 1–2.

5. No mention was made of the home visitors' race, but they were employed professionals, and it is reasonable to assume they were white since, particularly in Tennessee during the 1960s, employing African American professionals would have merited comment. Furthermore, Gray and her colleagues specifically mentioned that the classroom teaching staff was integrated. In the 1970s, Gray launched experimental programs in which the African American mothers who had participated in the intervention received training to serve as home visitors in future programs (Gray et al., *Before First Grade*, 2; Susan Gray, "Home Visiting Programs for Parents of Young Children," in *Emerging Strategies in Early Childhood Education*, ed. J. Wesley Little and Arthur J. Brigham [New York: MSS Information, 1973], 214–15).

6. Gray et al., *Before First Grade*, 103.

7. Edward Zigler and Jeanette Valentine, eds., *Project Head Start: A Legacy of the War on Poverty* (New York: Free Press, 1979), 10.

8. Dale Harris, "Early Experimental Deprivation and Enrichment and Later Development: An Introduction to a Symposium," *Child Development* 36, no. 4 (1965): 839–42.

9. "Study Emphasizes How Slums Retard Learning," *New York Times*, December 30, 1964.

10. Gray and Klaus, "Experimental Preschool Program," 888–89.

11. Susan Gray and Rupert Klaus, "Brief Reflections on the Theory of Early Childhood Enrichment Programs," in *Early Education: Current Theory, Research, and Action*, ed. Robert Hess and Roberta Bear (Chicago: Aldine, 1968), 67–68.

12. Gray and Klaus, "Experimental Preschool Program," 890.

13. Zigler and Styfco, *Hidden History*, 6–9.

14. Vinovskis, *Birth of Head Start*, 110–12.

15. Gray et al., *Before First Grade*, 22–23.

16. Ibid.

17. Ibid., 107–8.

18. Martin Deutsch, *Memorandum on Facilities for Early Childhood Education: Institute for Developmental Studies* (New York: Educational Facilities Laboratory, 1968), vi.

19. Ibid., 3–4.

20. Barbara Beatty, "The Debate over the Young 'Disadvantaged Child': Preschool Intervention, Developmental Psychology, and Compensatory Education in the 1960s and Early 1970s," *Teachers College Record* 114, no. 6 (2012): 1–36; Anahad O'Connor, "Dr. Martin Deutsch, an Innovator in Education, Dies at 76," *New York Times*, July 5, 2002.

21. For example, a 1968 report on the IDS preschool program makes no mention of race: The children are described as coming from "tenement homes that are economically, socially and culturally deprived." Perhaps the only description hinting at race is a quote from a little boy who spoke in nonstandard English (Martin Deutsch and the IDS Staff, *The Deutsch Model: Institute for Developmental Studies* [New York: New York University Institute for Developmental Studies, 1968], 1, 11).

22. Powledge, *To Change a Child*, 7–20.

23. Ibid., 52.

24. Martin Deutsch, "The Disadvantaged Child and the Learning Process," in *Education in Depressed Areas*, ed. Harry Passow (New York: Teachers College, Columbia University, 1963), 170.

25. Ibid., 176.

26. Martin Deutsch, "Nursery Education: The Influence of Social Programming on Early Development," in *The Disadvantaged Child: Selected Papers of Martin Deutsch and Associates*, ed. Martin Deutsch (New York: Basic Books, 1967), 68–69.

27. Cynthia Deutsch, "Environment and Perception," in *Social Class, Race, and Psychological Development*, ed. Martin Deutsch, Irwin Katz, and Arthur Jensen (New York: Holt, Rinehart, and Winston, 1968), 59.

28. Ibid., 80–83.

29. Martin Deutsch, *Memorandum on Facilities*, 9–10.

30. Martin Deutsch, *Deutsch Model*, 6–7, 16.

31. Ibid., 8.

32. Ibid.; Powledge, *To Change a Child*, 50.

33. Martin Deutsch, *Deutsch Model*, 8.

34. Ibid., 11.

35. Silberman had corresponded and met with Hunt while preparing reports on "new developments" in education (Dorothy Ferenbaugh to JMH, January 23, 1964, box 51, folder "Preschool Enrichment and Cultural Deprivation," JMH Papers).

36. Charles Silberman, *Crisis in Black and White* (New York: Vintage, 1964), 270–71. See also Margalit Fox, "Charles E. Silberman, Who Wrote about Racism in the U.S., Dies at 86," *New York Times*, February 13, 2011.

37. Silberman, *Crisis in Black and White*, 277.

38. Silberman, "Give Slum Children a Chance: A Radical Proposal," *Harper's Magazine*, May 1964, 37–42; Vinovskis, *Birth of Head Start*, 50–52. See also Beatty, "Debate," 9.

39. Powledge, *To Change a Child*, 74.

40. Fredric Wertham, *Seduction of the Innocent* (New York: Rinehart, 1954); David J. Pittman, "Mass Media and Juvenile Delinquency," in *Juvenile Delinquency*, ed. Joseph

Rouček (New York: Philosophical Library, 1958), 230–50; James Gilbert, *Cycle of Outrage: America's Reaction to the Juvenile Delinquent in the 1950s* (Oxford: Oxford University Press, 1986), 91–108.

41. Arnold Binder and Susan L. Polan, "The Kennedy-Johnson Years, Social Theory, and Federal Policy in the Control of Juvenile Delinquency," *Crime and Delinquency* 37, no. 2 (1991): 242–61; Gerald Markowitz and David Rosner, *Children, Race, and Power: Kenneth and Mamie Clark's Northside Center* (Charlottesville: University Press of Virginia, 1996), 186–89.

42. Barry C. Feld, *Bad Kids: Race and the Transformation of the Juvenile Court* (New York: Oxford University Press, 1999); Barry C. Feld, "Race and the Jurisprudence of Juvenile Justice: A Tale in Two Parts, 1950–2000," in *Our Children, Their Children: Confronting Racial and Ethnic Differences in American Juvenile Justice*, ed. Kimberly Kempf-Leonard and Darnell F. Hawkins (Chicago: University of Chicago Press, 2010), 122–63; Everette B. Penn, Helen Taylor Greene, and Shaun L. Gabbidon, eds., *Race and Juvenile Justice* (Durham: Carolina Academic Press, 2005); Michelle Alexander, *The New Jim Crow: Mass Incarceration in the Age of Colorblindness* (New York: New Press, 2010).

43. Cited in Jason Barnosky, "The Violent Years: Responses to Juvenile Crime in the 1950s," *Polity* 38, no. 3 (2006): 327.

44. Elizabeth A. Wells, *West Side Story: Cultural Perspectives on an American Musical* (Lanham, Md.: Scarecrow, 2011), 189–216, 263–65.

45. Barnosky, "Violent Years," 316–17.

46. Ibid., 332–33.

47. Sociologist Noel Cazenave has examined the success of the War on Poverty community action programs, focusing specifically on the MFY. This work is the most comprehensive analysis of these community action programs published to date; many of the earlier accounts were written during the period of the programs' activities, usually by persons involved in their inception. See Noel Cazenave, *Impossible Democracy: The Unlikely Success of the War on Poverty Community Action Programs* (Albany: SUNY Press, 2007). To illustrate, one edited volume on the educational and employment services at the MFY is dedicated to Winslow Carlton, chair of the MFY board. Sociologists Peter Marris and Martin Rein, who wrote an account of community action programs in the United States, were commissioned by the Ford Foundation and the President's Committee on Juvenile Delinquency, respectively, to observe the projects. See Harold H. Weissman, ed., *Employment and Educational Services in the Mobilization for Youth Experience* (New York: Association, 1969); Peter Marris and Martin Rein, *Dilemmas of Social Reform: Poverty and Community Action in the United States* (London: Routledge, 1972), 2–3. Prior to Cazenave's publication, the most authoritative account of the MFY experience was Joseph Helfgot, *Professional Reforming: Mobilization for Youth and the Failure of Social Science* (Lexington, Mass.: Lexington Books, 1981).

48. Moynihan describes the similarities between the MFY program and Johnson's War on Poverty, comparing the MFY's educational programs to Project Head Start (*Maximum Feasible Misunderstanding*, 54–59).

49. Richard Cloward and Lloyd Ohlin, *Delinquency and Opportunity: A Theory of Delinquent Gangs* (New York: Free Press, 1960); Alice O'Connor, *Poverty Knowledge:*

Social Science, Social Policy, and the Poor in Twentieth-Century U.S. History (Princeton: Princeton University Press, 2001), 124–35; Gilbert, *Cycle of Outrage*, 139–42; Markowitz and Rosner, *Children, Race, and Power*, 186–87; Vinovskis, *Birth of Head Start*, 29–32.

50. Harold Silver and Pamela Silver, *An Educational War on Poverty* (Cambridge: Cambridge University Press, 1991), 46.

51. Marjorie Martus, "The Special Case of the Young Disadvantaged Child," 1964, 4, Report 010351, Ford Foundation Records, Rockefeller Foundation Archives, Sleepy Hollow, N.Y.

52. Ibid., 11.

53. Marjorie Martus, "Early Childhood Education: A Background Paper," May 1965, 9, 41–43, Report 012573, Ford Foundation Records.

54. George Brager, "Some Assumptions and Strategies of the MFY Program," September 1962, box 24, folder "MFY Reports by MFY Members," Mobilization for Youth Records, Rare Book and Manuscript Library, Columbia University, New York.

55. Mobilization for Youth, *A Proposal for the Prevention and Control of Delinquency by Expanding Opportunities* (New York: Mobilization for Youth, 1961).

56. Cazenave, *Impossible Democracy*, 27. Opportunity theory was used even at times when it seemed quite a stretch, such as an attempt to interpret delinquency in young women as resulting from a lack of appropriate opportunities for marriage and social development (Mobilization for Youth, *Proposal*, 52–54).

57. Cazenave, *Impossible Democracy*, 69–75; Alice O'Connor, *Poverty Knowledge*, 127–34.

58. Joseph Helfgot, "Professional Reform Organizations and the Symbolic Representation of the Poor," *American Sociological Review* 39, no. 4 (1974): 475–91.

59. Ibid., 490.

60. Lillian B. Rubin, "Maximum Feasible Participation: The Origins, Implications, and Present Status," *Annals of the American Academy of Political and Social Science* 385, no. 1 (1969): 14–29; Moynihan, *Maximum Feasible Misunderstanding*, 54–59; Alice O'Connor, *Poverty Knowledge*, 171–82; Tara J. Melish, "Maximum Feasible Participation of the Poor: New Governance, New Accountability, and a 21st Century War on the Sources of Poverty," *Yale Human Rights and Development Law Journal* 13, no. 1 (2010): 1–130.

61. Both major accounts of the MFY project address the coexistence of a "culture of poverty" approach alongside the opportunity theory, yet neither refers specifically to the use of deprivation theories (Helfgot, *Professional Reforming*, 44–48, 54–55; Cazenave, *Impossible Democracy*, 97).

62. Mobilization for Youth, *Proposal*, 73.

63. Ibid., 74.

64. Ibid., 111.

65. Ibid., 107–8.

66. Ibid., 115.

67. See also A. Harry Passow, "Urban Education: The New Challenge," *Educational Researcher* 6, no. 9 (1977): 5–10; Cazenave, *Impossible Democracy*, 74–83.

68. Mobilization for Youth, *Proposal*, 306.

69. Ibid., 121, 307 (the same outline appears twice in the proposal).

70. Minutes of Board of Directors Meeting, April 10, 1963, 8, box 3, folder 2, Mobilization for Youth Records; Mobilization for Youth, *Proposal*, 108, 278; Mobilization for Youth, *Action on the Lower East Side: Progress Report and Proposal* (New York: Mobilization for Youth, 1966), 43.

71. "MFY World of Education Summary Report, September 1962–September 1964," 16, box 7, folder "Committee on Educational Opportunity Orientation Materials," Mobilization for Youth Records.

72. Sandra I. Kay, "An Interview with Abraham J. Tannenbaum: Innovative Programs for the Gifted and Talented," *Roeper Review* 24, no. 4 (2002): 186.

73. "MFY World of Education—Plans for MFY Reading Program 1965–66," March 15, 1965, 4, box 7, folder "Committee on Educational Opportunity Orientation Materials," Mobilization for Youth Records.

74. Abraham J. Tannenbaum, "MFY in NYC," May 1966, 6, box 16, folder "MFY Committee on Educational Opportunities Meetings and Reports, 1966," John H. Niemeyer Papers, Bank Street College of Education, Record Group 2, Subgroup 2, Series H, New York.

75. Ibid.

76. Minutes of Meeting, Committee on Educational Opportunities, June 27, 1966, 1, box 16, folder "MFY Committee on Educational Opportunities Meetings and Reports, 1966," Niemeyer Papers.

77. "Second Draft Proposal for a Laboratory Pre School in an Urban Depressed Area," April 15, 1966, 3, 7, box 16, folder "MFY Committee on Educational Opportunities—Meetings and Reports, 1966," Niemeyer Papers.

78. Abraham J. Tannenbaum, "An Evaluation of STAR, or the Effects of Training and Deputizing Indigenous Adults to Administer a Home-Based Tutoring Program to First Graders in an Urban Depressed Area," Mobilization for Youth, 1967, ERIC ED013852.

79. George Brager, "The Low Income Nonprofessional," in *Community Action against Poverty: Readings from the Mobilization Experience*, ed. George Brager and Francis Purcell (New Haven: College and University Press, 1967), 163–74; Helfgot, *Professional Reforming*, 158–69.

80. Tannenbaum, "Evaluation of STAR," 28–29.

81. "Herbert Burton Goldsmith: Obituary," *New York Times*, March 4, 2008.

82. Herbert Goldsmith to Jane Lee Eddy, April 5, 1967, box 16, folder "MFY Committee on Educational Opportunities: Meetings and Reports, 1967," Niemeyer Papers.

83. *A School Orientation Program for Parents*, n.d., box 16, folder "MFY Committee on Educational Opportunities: Meetings and Reports, 1967," Niemeyer Papers.

84. Abraham J. Tannenbaum, "Evaluating STAR: Non-Professional Tutoring," *Teachers College Record* 69, no. 5 (1958): 446.

85. McCandish Philips, "Youths to Picket Job Center Today," *New York Times*, May 8, 1963; Martin Tolchin, "Project's Road Has Been Rocky," *New York Times*, August 17, 1964; Powledge, "Mobilization for Youth."

86. Albert Fried, "The Attack on Mobilization," in *Community Development in the Mobilization for Youth Experience*, ed. Harold Weissman (New York: Association, 1969), 137–38.

87. Michael Reisch and Janice Andrews, *The Road Not Taken: A History of Radical*

Social Work in the United States (New York: Brunner-Routledge, 2002), 142–44; William M. Epstein, *Democracy without Decency: Good Citizenship and the War on Poverty* (University Park: Pennsylvania State University Press, 2010), 31–34.

88. Helfgot, *Professional Reforming*, 88–102; Cazenave, *Impossible Democracy*, 118–23; Moynihan, *Maximum Feasible Misunderstanding*, 102–3.

89. Cazenave, *Impossible Democracy*, 116–36; Fried, "Attack on Mobilization," 137–48.

90. Harlem Youth Opportunities Unlimited, *Youth in the Ghetto: A Study of the Consequences of Powerlessness and a Blueprint for Change* (New York: Harlem Youth Opportunities Unlimited, 1964), 22; Kenneth Clark, Interview by Ed Edwin, Session 4, April 7, 1976, 147, Columbia University Center for Oral History, New York; Markowitz and Rosner, *Children, Race, and Power*, 188–200; Cazenave, *Impossible Democracy*, 87–88.

91. Clark, Interview, 147–49. See also Ben Keppel, *The Work of Democracy: Ralph Bunche, Kenneth B. Clark, Lorraine Hansberry, and the Cultural Politics of Race* (Cambridge: Harvard University Press, 1995), 133–77; Markowitz and Rosner, *Children, Race, and Power*, 79–82, 189; Cheryl Lynn Greenberg, *Troubling the Waters: Black-Jewish Relations in the American Century* (Princeton: Princeton University Press, 2006).

92. Cazenave, *Impossible Democracy*, 96–97.

93. Ibid., 85–104; Alice O'Connor, *Poverty Knowledge*, 201–2.

94. Harlem Youth Opportunities Unlimited, *Youth in the Ghetto*, 287–89; Cazenave, *Impossible Democracy*, 96–99.

95. Harlem Youth Opportunities Unlimited, *Youth in the Ghetto*, 199. The source for the description of this child is not cited.

96. Ibid., 206–17, 239.

97. For a comprehensive analysis of Project Head Start, see Vinovskis, *Birth of Head Start*. Primary material can be found in Zigler and Valentine, *Project Head Start*; Edward Zigler and Susan Muenchow, *Head Start: The Inside Story of America's Most Successful Educational Experiment* (New York: Basic Books, 1992). For a historical analysis from an insider's perspective, see Zigler and Styfco, *Hidden History*.

98. Diane Ravitch, *The Troubled Crusade: American Education, 1945–1980* (New York: Basic Books, 1983), 159–60; Zigler and Styfco, *Hidden History*, 57.

99. Vinovskis, *Birth of Head Start*, 76–82; Zigler and Styfco, *Hidden History*, 59–62.

100. Vinovskis, *Birth of Head Start*, 149–52.

101. Zigler and Styfco, *Hidden History*, 56–60; OEO, "A Prospectus on Early Childhood Development for the Children of the Poor," January 21, 1965, box 16, folder 21, Urie Bronfenbrenner Papers, 23-13-954, Division of Rare and Manuscript Collections, Cornell University Library, Ithaca, N.Y.

102. Sargent Shriver to Urie Bronfenbrenner, February 19, 1965, box 16, folder 21, Bronfenbrenner Papers.

103. In 1966, psychologist Urie Bronfenbrenner described Project Head Start as the "first attack on a national scale against the devastating effects of cultural deprivation in infancy" ("Institutional Approaches to Cultural Deprivation—American and Soviet," paper presented at the Third International Scientific Symposium on Mental Retardation, Boston, April 11, 1966, box 9, folder 40, Bronfenbrenner Papers).

104. JBR to Edward T. Wakemen, February 22, 1966, box 9, folder 23, JBR Papers. In June 1967, Richmond argued at an OEO meeting that the prevention of nutritional de-

ficiencies was one of the most important contributions of Project Head Start (Minutes of OEO Meeting, June 1967, box 26, folder 13, JBR Papers). See, for example, David K. Silver to JBR, July 13, 1965, box 26, folder 7, JBR Papers (offering the National Vitamin Foundation's assistance).

105. Zigler and Styfco, *Hidden History*, 3–87; Vinovskis, *Birth of Head Start*, 60–86. The relationship between certain nutritional deficiencies and learning ability was the focus of much research. See, for example, Nancy Munro, *The Relationship between Hemoglobin Level and Intellectual Function* (Missoula: Montana University Foundation, 1967).

106. Zigler and Styfco, *Hidden History*, 94–95.

107. For example, in 1967, senior Head Start pediatrician Frederick North wrote to psychiatrist Barbara Munk that he could "find no evidence that the mental health professions brought different perspectives or skills to the observations" (Frederick North to Barbara Munk, March 8, 1967, Group for the Advancement of Psychiatry Papers, box 14, folder 2, Oskar Diethelm Library, Weill Medical College Institute for the History of Psychiatry, Cornell University, New York).

108. U.S. Department of Agriculture, *Project Head Start: Food Buying Guide and Recipes* (Washington, D.C.: U.S. Office of Economic Opportunity, 1967); U.S. Department of Agriculture, Nutrition Programs Service Unit, *Proceedings of Nutrition Education Conference, February 20–22, 1967* (Washington, D.C.: U.S. Department of Agriculture, 1968).

109. Jean Murphy, "Learn to Eat: Children in Head Start on Nutrition," *Los Angeles Times*, October 26, 1967; "Head Start to Sponsor Nutrition Conference," *Los Angeles Times*, November 9, 1967; Rose Dosti, "Head Start Nutrition Project Teaching Children Diet Value," *Los Angeles Times*, April 3, 1969.

110. Luise K. Addiss, *Jenny Is a Good Thing* (Washington, D.C.: U.S. Department of Health, Education, and Welfare, 1969); "Specialist Works with Head Start," *Los Angeles Times*, August 15, 1968.

111. Jean Murphy, "Learn to Eat"; Eve Jensen, "Where Operation Head Start Begins Best—With the Tummy," *Los Angeles Times*, August 11, 1966.

112. OEO, "Early Childhood Programs," 11, March 18, 1965, box 18, JBR Papers.

113. OEO, "Improving the Opportunities and Achievements of the Children of the Poor," February 1965, box 58, folder "Head Start, 1965–66," JMH Papers.

114. Cited in Vinovskis, *Birth of Head Start*, 88; Zigler and Styfco, *Hidden History*, 35.

115. David McL. Greeley to JBR, April 22, 1965, box 26, folder 7, JBR Papers.

116. JBR to JMH, May 5, 1965, box 58, folder "Head Start, 1965–66," JMH Papers.

117. JMH to JBR, May 23, 1965, box 58, folder "Head Start, 1965–66," JMH Papers.

118. JBR to JMH, June 8, 1965, box 58, folder "Head Start, 1965–66," JMH Papers.

119. Glendon P. Nimnicht, Oralie McAfee, and John H. Meier, *The New Nursery School* (New York: General Learning Corporation, 1969), 4; "Unlocking Early Learning Secrets," *Life*, March 31, 1967.

120. John H. Meier, Glendon P. Nimnicht, and Oralie McAfee, "An Autotelic Responsive Environment Nursery School for Deprived Children," in *Disadvantaged Child*, vol. 2, *Head Start and Early Intervention*, ed. Jerome Hellmuth (New York: Brunner/Mazal, 1968), 299–398. The article they cite is Mark Rosenzweig, "Environmental Complexity, Cerebral Change, and Behavior," *American Psychologist* 21, no. 4 (1966): 321–32.

121. Meier, Nimnicht, and McAfee, "Autotelic Responsive Environment," 308–9.

122. Ibid., 329.

123. "Glendon Nimnicht, Ed.D., Recipient, Kellogg's Child Development Award," http://www.worldofchildren.org/honorees/2002–honorees/82–glendon-nimnicht.

124. Eveline Omwake, "Head Start—Measurable and Immeasurable," in *Disadvantaged Child*, ed. Hellmuth, 2:531–44; Vinovskis, *Birth of Head Start*, 87–118.

125. Edward Zigler and Penelope Trickett, "IQ, Social Competence, and Evaluation of Early Childhood Intervention Programs," *American Psychologist* 33, no. 9 (1978): 789–98; Ravitch, *Troubled Crusade*, 159; Alice O'Connor, *Poverty Knowledge*, 185–90; Zigler and Styfco, *Hidden History*, 68–85, 179–201.

126. Powledge, *To Change a Child*, 6; Zigler and Styfco, *Hidden History*, 100–104.

127. James Samuel Coleman, *Equality of Educational Opportunity* (Washington, D.C.: U.S. Department of Health, Education, and Welfare, 1966); *Racial Isolation in the Public Schools* (Washington, D.C.: U.S. Government Printing Office, 1967).

128. Although the findings of the Coleman Report were not clear-cut, and in certain conditions, children in all-black schools outperformed their peers in desegregated settings, the idea that racial integration was the magic bullet for improving African American achievement was rapidly disseminated. At the same time, Coleman confided in some colleagues that his findings suggested that school education was too late and that early intervention was in fact the key (Ravitch, *Troubled Crusade*, 170–72). In a 1967 letter to Daniel Patrick Moynihan, Coleman suggested replacing the environment of young African American children, proposing "things like daytime group homes, with plenty of middle-class white mothers around, for very young children," demonstrating again the interrelations between theories of environmental deprivation and maternal deprivation (cited in James T. Patterson, *Freedom Is Not Enough: The Moynihan Report and America's Struggle over Black Family Life from LBJ to Obama* [New York: Basic Books, 2010], 104).

129. Ravitch, *Troubled Crusade*, 168–75.

130. Kevin L. Yull, "The 1966 White House Conference on Civil Rights," *Historical Journal* 41, no. 1 (1998): 275.

131. Edward Zigler and Winnie Berman, "Discerning the Future of Early Childhood Intervention," *American Psychologist* 38, no. 8 (1983): 894; Edward Zigler, "Formal Schooling for Four-Year-Olds?: No," *American Psychologist* 42, no. 3 (1987): 258; Edward Zigler and Sally Styfco, "Head Start: Criticisms in a Constructive Context," *American Psychologist* 49, no. 2 (1994): 127–32.

132. Edward Zigler, "Reshaping Early Childhood Intervention to Be a More Effective Weapon against Poverty," *American Journal of Community Psychology* 22, no. 1 (1994): 40–41; Charles Locurto, "Beyond IQ in Preschool Programs," *Intelligence* 15, no. 3 (1991): 295–312; Charles Locurto, "Hands on the Elephant: IQ, Preschool Programs, and the Rhetoric of Inoculation: A Reply to Commentaries," *Intelligence* 15, no. 3 (1991): 335–49. For a few examples of citations of Zigler, see Jeanne Brooks-Gunn, "Strategies for Altering the Outcomes of Poor Children and their Families," in *Escape from Poverty: What Makes a Difference for Children?*, ed. P. Lindsay Chase-Lansdale and Jeanne Brooks-Gunn (New York: Cambridge University Press, 1995), 100; George S. Baroff and J. Gregory Olley, *Mental Retardation: Nature, Cause, and Management* (Phila-

delphia: Taylor and Francis, 1999), 228; Sheldon H. White and Deborah A. Phillips, "Designing Head Start: Roles Played by Developmental Psychologists," in *Social Science and Policy-Making: A Search for Relevance in the Twentieth Century*, ed. David Featherman and Maris A. Vinovskis (Ann Arbor: University of Michigan Press, 2001), 96–100. In an encyclopedia entry on Head Start, Sally Styfco referred to the "then-popular 'inoculation model'" ("Head Start," in *The Concise Corsini Encyclopedia of Psychology and Behavioral Science*, 3rd ed., ed. W. Edward Craighead and Charles B. Nemeroff [Hoboken, N.J.: Wiley, 2004], 428).

133. James Colgrove, *State of Immunity: The Politics of Vaccination in Twentieth Century America* (Berkeley: University of California Press, 2006), 149–85.

134. Ibid., 161–62. For data concerning children's access to health care prior to Head Start, see Zigler and Styfco, *Hidden History*, 123.

135. Richard Orton, national director of the Head Start program, was cited as saying, "Head Start never was intended as a one-shot inoculation that would save the child for the rest of his life" (John Herber, "Director Defends Head Start's Work; Says It Aids Pupils," *New York Times*, April 15, 1969).

136. Leon Eisenberg and C. Keith Conners, "The Effect of Head Start on Developmental Processes," paper presented at the Joseph P. Kennedy Jr. Symposium on Mental Retardation, April 11, 1966, Boston, ERIC ED020026. This statement was also cited in a newspaper article, "Headstart Gains Lauded by Hopkins Psychologist," *Baltimore Sun*, April 12, 1966.

137. Hilliard E. Chesteen Jr., "Effectiveness of the Head Start Program in Enhancing School Readiness of Culturally Deprived Children," 47–50, 144–46, Community Advancement, Baton Rouge, 1966, ERIC ED020771.

138. Ibid., 150–51.

139. Ibid., 156–57.

140. Westinghouse Learning Corporation, *The Impact of Head Start* (Washington, D.C.: U.S. Department of Health Education and Welfare, 1969).

141. Robert B. Semple Jr., "White House and Advisers Stand by Report Critical of Head Start Program," *New York Times*, April 27, 1969.

142. Fred M. Hechinger, "Dispute over Value of Head Start," *New York Times*, April 20, 1969; M. A. Farber, "Head Start Report Held 'Full of Holes': Head Start Report Assailed as 'Full of Holes' and Potential Political Disaster," *New York Times*, April 18, 1969.

143. William G. Madow to John W. Evans, March 18, 1969, box 27, folder 3, JBR Papers; Edward Zigler to Daniel P. Moynihan, March 25, 1969, box 27, folder 3, JBR Papers. Richmond termed the report a "disaster" and said that it would have been "funny" had it not been "malicious" (JBR to Urie Bronfenbrenner, April 16, 1969, box 7, folder 2, JBR Papers). See also Nancie Stewart and Marjorie Grosett, "Programs for Deprived Children—Letter to the Editor," *New York Times*, May 3, 1969.

144. Zigler and Styfco, *Hidden History*, 179–84.

145. Sheldon White, "Comments on the Preliminary Draft of the 'Impact of Headstart,'" enclosed with letter to Daniel P. Moynihan, March 26, 1969, box 27, folder 3, JBR Papers.

146. Zigler and Styfco, *Hidden History*, 83; Jeaneda H. Nolan, "A Report on the Evaluation of the State Preschool Program Contrasted with the Westinghouse Report on

Head Start," edited transcript of a speech to the State Board of Education, Sacramento, Calif., June 12, 1969, ERIC ED039920.

147. Zigler and Trickett, "IQ, Social Competence, and Evaluation."

148. Sylvia L. M. Martinez and John L. Rury, "From 'Culturally Deprived' to 'At Risk': The Politics of Popular Expression and Educational Inequality in the United States, 1960–1985," *Teachers College Record* 114, no. 6 (2012): 8–15.

149. *Head Start Amendments of 1998*, July 16, 1998, 105th Congress, H.R. 4241; Zigler and Styfco, *Hidden History*, 148–49, 282–84.

150. An analysis of data from 1965 found that African American children from metropolitan areas were 6.97 times more likely than their white counterparts to participate in Head Start; in nonmetropolitan areas, this ratio was 4.77 (Coleman, *Equality of Educational Opportunity*, 492). According to Zigler, the program faced accusations of discrimination because it served a disproportionately low number of white children (Zigler and Styfco, *Hidden History*, 95, 126–27).

151. David Carter, *The Music Has Gone Out of the Movement: Civil Rights and the Johnson Administration, 1965–1968* (Chapel Hill: University of North Carolina Press, 2009), 31–50, 103–32; Kimberly Morgan, "A Child of the Sixties: The Great Society, the New Right, and the Politics of Federal Child Care," *Journal of Policy History* 13, no. 2 (2001): 226–27; Erica Duncan, "Long after '65, Still Fighting to Overcome," *New York Times*, September 10, 1995; John Dittmer, *The Good Doctors: The Medical Committee for Human Rights and the Struggle for Social Justice in Health Care* (New York: Bloomsbury, 2009,) 125–27. For a history of Head Start and the Child Development Group of Mississippi written by a participant and activist, see Polly Greenberg, *The Devil Has Slippery Shoes* (New York: Macmillan, 1969). See also Zigler and Styfco, *Hidden History*, 126.

152. Kenneth Clark, "Alternative Public School Systems—A Response to America's Educational Emergency," 6–7, paper presented at the U.S. Conference on Civil Rights, November 16–17, 1967, Washington D.C., ERIC ED015981.

153. Ravitch, *Troubled Crusade*, 153.

CHAPTER FOUR

1. Throughout this chapter I use in quotation marks the term common at the time, "mental retardation," exclusively when referring to contemporary debates and publications. The currently accepted term, "intellectual disability," will be used when providing historiographic background or analysis. While the concept of intellectual disability has replaced that of mental retardation, there is no clear continuity between the two categories. It is likely that many of the children referred to as "mildly mentally retarded" in the texts examined in this chapter would not be diagnosed today with intellectual disability. Thus, throughout the text, I use the term "mild mental retardation" in quotation marks. See Robert L. Schalock, Ruth A. Luckasson, and Karrie A. Shogren, "The Renaming of Mental Retardation: Understanding the Change to the Term 'Intellectual Disability,'" *Intellectual and Developmental Disabilities* 45, no. 2 (2007): 116–24.

2. Beth Harry and Janette Klingner, *Why Are So Many Minority Students in Special Education?: Understanding Race and Disability in Schools* (New York: Teachers College Press, 2006), 2–6; Suzanne Donovan and Christopher T. Cross, eds., *Minority Students*

in Special and Gifted Education (Washington, D.C.: National Academies Press, 2002), 36–38.

3. Beth Ferri and David Connor, "Tools of Exclusion: Race, Disability and (Re)segregated Education," *Teachers College Record* 107, no. 3 (2005): 458; Wanda Blanchett, "Disproportionate Representation of African American Students in Special Education: Acknowledging the Role of White Privilege and Racism," *Educational Researcher* 35, no. 6 (2006): 25–26.

4. Christine Sleeter, "Learning Disabilities: The Social Construction of a Special Education Category," *Exceptional Children* 53, no. 1 (1986): 46–54; Wanda Blanchett, Vincent Mumford, and Floyd Beachum, "Urban School Failure and Disproportionality in a Post-*Brown* Era," *Remedial and Special Education* 26, no. 2 (2005): 70–81; Beth Ferri and David Connor, "In the Shadow of *Brown*: Special Education and Overrepresentation of Students of Color," *Remedial and Special Educational* 26, no. 2 (2005): 93–100.

5. Edward Zigler and Robert M. Hodapp, *Understanding Mental Retardation* (Cambridge: Cambridge University Press, 1986), 3.

6. Arthur L. Benton, "Psychological Evaluation and Differential Diagnosis," in *Mental Retardation*, ed. Harvey A. Stevens and Rick F. Heber (Chicago: University of Chicago Press, 1964), 45.

7. Richard Heber, "Terminology and the Classification of Mental Retardation," *American Journal of Mental Deficiency*, suppl. 64, no. 2 (1959): 1–111. Apart from the introduction of the concept of "adaptive behavior," the classifications are nearly identical, and I refer to the earlier publication. For a further evaluation of the concept of adaptive behavior, see Stephen Greenspan and Harvey N. Switzky, "Forty-Four Years of AAMR Manuals," in *What Is Mental Retardation?: Ideas for an Evolving Disability in the 21st Century*, ed. Harvey N. Switzky and Stephen Greenspan (Washington, D.C.: American Association on Mental Retardation, 2006), 3–28; George S. Baroff, "On the 2002 AAMR Definition of Mental Retardation," in *What Is Mental Retardation?*, ed. Switzky and Greenspan, 29–38.

8. Herbert J. Grossman, ed., *Manual on Terminology and Classification in Mental Retardation* (Washington, D.C.: American Association on Mental Deficiency, 1973), 11.

9. Heber, "Terminology," 8–9.

10. Ibid., 39–40.

11. Indeed, the glossary lists only one form of deprivation, "deprivation, environmental," and defines it as "reductions or lacks in environmental stimulation and in opportunities for acquiring knowledge ordinarily provided young children" (Heber, "Terminology," 90).

12. The *DSM II* classification was revised to follow and "incorporate AAMD concepts," according to participants at the Committee on Nomenclature and Statistics meeting, December 19, 1966, American Psychiatric Association Board of Trustees Files, box 100223, folder 223, Melvin Sabshin Library and Archives, American Psychiatric Association, Alexandria, Va.

Although nearly a decade after the appearance of the 1959 *AAMD Manual*, the incorporation of the concept of deprivation into the *ICD 8* was still the subject of controversy. It was ultimately resolved following the recommendations of two experts, American psychiatrist Henry Brill and A. V. Snezhnevsky, director of the Soviet Union's

Institute of Psychiatry of the Academy of Medical Sciences, who were asked to comment on three controversial diagnoses: antisocial personality, reactive psychosis, and mental retardation with psychosocial deprivation. While their recommendations are not noted in the text and no minutes of these discussions are available, the ultimate result was the acceptance of the diagnosis of psychosocial deprivation. See Iwao Milton Moriyama, "The Eighth Revision of the International Classification of Diseases," *American Journal of Public Health and the Nation's Health* 56, no. 8 (1966): 1279. This acceptance is not surprising in light of reports such as those of Harold Skeels, a psychologist and expert on intellectual disability who had participated more than a decade earlier in the World Health Organization's Expert Committee on the Mentally Defective Child. Skeels described the members' "willing acceptance" of deprivation alone, without any biological predisposition, as a sufficient cause of intellectual deficiency, thus forgoing previous heredity-based approaches (Harold Skeels, "Report on World Health Organization Expert Committee on the Mentally Defective Child and Visits in London," report presented at the NIMH General Staff Meeting, March 1953, box M50, folder Harold Skeels, Archives of the History of American Psychology, Center for the History of Psychology, University of Akron, Akron, Ohio).

13. Robert Spitzer and Paul T. Wilson, "A Guide to the American Psychiatric Association's New Diagnostic Nomenclature," *American Journal of Psychiatry* 124, no. 12 (1968): 1625.

14. American Psychiatric Association, *Diagnostic and Statistical Manual of Mental Disorders*, 2nd ed. (Washington, D.C.: American Psychiatric Association, 1968), 21.

15. Ibid., 22.

16. Paul T. Wilson and Robert Spitzer, "A Comparison of Three Current Classification Systems for Mental Retardation," *American Journal of Mental Deficiency* 74, no. 3 (1969): 435.

17. Howard Potter, "Mental Retardation: The Cinderella of Psychiatry," *Psychiatric Quarterly* 39, no. 1 (1965): 537–48; Edward Davens, interview by John Stewart, March 29, 1968, 1–5, John F. Kennedy Library Oral History Program, Boston.

18. James Trent, *Inventing the Feeble Mind: A History of Mental Retardation in the United States* (Berkeley: University of California Press, 1994), 230–34; Robert Osgood, *The History of Inclusion in the United States* (Washington, D.C.: Gallaudet University Press, 2005), 56–59; Michael Grossberg, "From Feeble-Minded to Mentally Retarded: Child Protection and the Changing Place of Disabled Children in the Mid-Twentieth Century United States," *Paedagogica Historica* 47, no. 6 (2011): 729–47.

19. See Edward Berkowitz, "The Politics of Mental Retardation during the Kennedy Administration," *Social Science Quarterly* 61, no. 1 (1980): 130–33. Berkowitz describes how metaphors of the space race shaped the approach to "combating" intellectual disability.

20. Christine Sleeter, "Why Is There Learning Disabilities?: A Critical Analysis of the Birth of the Field in Its Social Context," in *The Formation of School Subjects: The Struggle for Creating an American Institution*, ed. Thomas S. Popkewitz (London: Palmer, 1987), 216.

21. Edith Asbury, "Rose Kennedy Tells of Her Retarded Daughter," *New York Times*, October 31, 1963.

22. For an in-depth analysis of the Kennedy family's role in the struggle for better care and treatment of persons with intellectual disabilities, see Edward Shorter, *The Kennedy Family and the Story of Mental Retardation* (Philadelphia: Temple University Press, 2000); Berkowitz, "Politics of Mental Retardation."

23. Shorter, *Kennedy Family*, 67–80.

24. John F. Kennedy, "Statement Regarding the Need for a National Plan in Mental Retardation," October 11, 1961, 1, http://www.mnddc.org/parallels2/pdf/60s/62/62-sallinger-pr.pdf. Edward Davens, a pediatrician and member of the President's Panel on Mental Retardation, specifically refers to the president's awareness of the detrimental effects of economic deprivation (interview, 6–7).

25. Lloyd Dunn and Samuel Kirk, "Impressions of Soviet Psycho-Educational Service and Research in Mental Retardation," *Exceptional Children* 29, no. 7 (1963): 301; "U.S. Scientists to Visit Red Mental Hospitals," *Washington Post*, June 1, 1962.

26. President's Panel on Mental Retardation, *A Proposed Program for National Action to Combat Mental Retardation* (Washington, D.C.: U.S. Government Printing Office, 1962), 8.

27. Robert P. Goldman, "5,600,000 of Us Are Mentally Retarded," *New York Times*, November 22, 1964.

28. President's Panel on Mental Retardation, *Proposed Program*, 61–62.

29. Ibid., 66–67.

30. Ibid., 67.

31. Ibid.

32. John F. Kennedy, "Message from the President of the United States Relative to Mental Illness and Mental Retardation, February 5, 1963," *Pastoral Psychology*, 15, no. 4 (1964): 15.

33. *Comments by Interested Individuals and Organizations on H.R. 3386, the Maternal and Child Health and Mental Retardation Planning Amendments of 1963* (Washington, D.C.: U.S. Government Printing Office, 1963). In fact, no unfavorable comments on the bill were sent to the committee (Berkowitz, "Politics of Mental Retardation," 139–40).

34. Lucy Ozarin and Steven Scharfstein, "The Aftermaths of Deinstitutionalization: Problems and Solutions," *Psychiatric Quarterly* 50, no. 2 (1978): 128–32; H. Richard Lamb, "Deinstitutionalization at the Beginning of a New Millennium," *Harvard Review of Psychiatry* 6, no. 1 (1998): 1–10; Gerald Grob, *The Mad among Us: A History of the Care of America's Mentally Ill* (New York: Free Press, 1994), 290–91; Jonathan Metzl, *The Protest Psychosis: How Schizophrenia Became a Black Disease* (Boston: Beacon, 2010), 131–36; Michael Staub, *Madness Is Civilization: When the Diagnosis Was Social, 1948–1980* (Chicago: University of Chicago Press, 2011), 183–88.

35. Group for the Advancement of Psychiatry, Committee on Mental Retardation, *Report No. 43: Basic Considerations in Mental Retardation: A Preliminary Report* (New York: GAP, 1959), 12.

36. Carl Scheckel to JMH, September 4, 1964, box 51, folder "Preschool Enrichment and Cultural Deprivation," JMH Papers.

37. Joseph Wortis, "Prevention of Mental Retardation," *American Journal of Orthopsychiatry* 35, no. 5 (1965): 889.

38. Burton Blatt, "A Concept of Educability and the Correlates of Mental Illness,

Mental Retardation, and Cultural Deprivation," in *Diminished People: Problems and Care of the Mentally Retarded*, ed. Norman Bernstein (Boston: Little, Brown, 1970), 16.

39. Edward M. Kennedy, preface to Rodger L. Hurley, *Poverty and Mental Retardation: A Causal Relationship* (New York: Vintage, 1969), xi.

40. Herbert Goldstein, *The Educable Mentally Retarded Child in the Elementary School* (Washington, D.C.: National Education Association, 1962), 12.

41. Group for the Advancement of Psychiatry, Committee on Mental Retardation, *Report No. 66, Mild Mental Retardation: A Growing Challenge to the Physician* (New York: GAP, 1967), 592.

42. Ibid., 596.

43. See, for example, Eric Avila, *Popular Culture in the Age of White Flight: Fear and Fantasy in Suburban Los Angeles* (Berkeley: University of California Press, 2004), 1–19.

44. "Insufficient or discontinuous mothering with physical neglect" was the first on a list of five "sociocultural factors" that characterized Group A children, including "distorted patterns of children rearing," disorganized families, social isolation, and conditions of poverty and crowding (Group for the Advancement of Psychiatry, Committee on Mental Retardation, *Report No. 66*, 614).

45. Ibid., 596.

46. Lois B. Murphy to Robert A. Haines, October 8, 1964, box M 1811, folder 10, G&LBM Papers.

47. Kansas Governor's Committee on Preschool Mental Retardation, Minutes of Meeting, February 11, 1965, 1, box 60, folder 1, Lois B. Murphy Papers, Modern Manuscripts Collection, History of Medicine Division, National Library of Medicine, Bethesda, Md., MS C 280c. See also, for example, R. K. Davenport Jr., E. W. Menzel Jr., and C. M Rogers, "Maternal Care during Infancy: Its Effect on Weight Gain and Mortality in the Chimpanzee," *American Journal of Orthopsychiatry* 31, no. 4 (1961): 803–9.

48. Lois B. Murphy, "Task Force I: Requirements of Infants for Normal Development in the First Year of Life," ca. early 1965, 3, box M1811, folder 10, G&LBM Papers.

49. Kansas Governor's Committee on Mental Retardation, "Task Force I, Preliminary Outline for a Program for Deprived Children," ca. early 1965, box M1811, folder 10, G&LBM Papers.

50. René A. Spitz, remarks at a conference on deprivation, draft, September 9, 1964, box M2124, folder 11, RAS Papers. Psychiatrist David A. Freedman, who had performed considerable research on the topic of sensory deprivation, examined the role of early mother-child relations in the etiology of mental retardation, relying on the analogy with sensory deprivation studies (David A. Freedman, "The Role of Early Mother/Child Relations in the Etiology of Some Cases of Mental Retardation," in *Congenital Mental Retardation*, ed. Gordon Farrell [Austin: University of Texas Press, 1969], 245–62).

51. Bowlby and Ainsworth claimed that studies of children in institutions had led researchers to understand the role of the parents in the etiology of mental retardation: "Parents who interact insufficiently with their children throughout the first few years of life" could cause damage comparable to that inflicted by life in "overcrowded, impersonal institutions" (John Bowlby and MA to the Joseph P. Kennedy Jr. Foundation, July 29, 1963, box M3176, folder 5, MA Papers).

52. In the 1963 *Handbook of Mental Deficiency*, one of the main reference books of the

time in the field of intellectual disability, a chapter titled "Sensory Processes and Mental Deficiency" examined the interface between sensory deprivation and mental retardation. Summarizing the early findings of sensory deprivation studies, the *Handbook*'s authors suggested that "mental retardation" operated in a manner similar to partial sensory deprivation (Frank Kodman, "Sensory Processes and Mental Deficiency," in *Handbook of Mental Deficiency*, ed. Norman Ellis [New York: McGraw-Hill, 1963], 471).

53. George Tarjan, "Sensory Deprivation and Mental Retardation," in *The Psychodynamic Implications of Physiological Studies on Sensory Deprivation*, ed. Leo Madow and Laurence Snow (Springfield, IL: Charles C. Thomas, 1970), 71.

54. Ibid., 73.

55. George Tarjan, "Some Thoughts on Sociocultural Retardation," in *Social-Cultural Aspects of Mental Retardation*, ed. H. Carl Haywood (New York: Appleton-Century-Crofts, 1970), 754. For a description of the significance of this conference, see Zigler and Hodapp, *Understanding Mental Retardation*, 80.

56. President's Committee on Mental Retardation, *A 1st Report to the President on the Nation's Progress and Remaining Great Needs in the Campaign to Combat Mental Retardation* (Washington, D.C.: President's Committee on Mental Retardation, 1967); President's Committee on Mental Retardation, *The Edge of Change: A Report to the President on Mental Retardation Program Trends and Innovations, with Recommendations on Residential Care, Manpower, and Deprivation* (Washington, D.C.: President's Committee on Mental Retardation, 1968), 24.

57. President's Committee on Mental Retardation, *Edge of Change*, 24.

58. Urie Bronfenbrenner to Michael Mansfield, Fred Harris, Russell Long, Robert F. Kennedy, and Jacob Javits, December 14, 1967, box 7, folder 2, JBR Papers.

59. Richard Koch, "Annual Presidential Message to the AAMD Membership," *American Journal of Mental Deficiency* 74, no. 1 (1969): 2–4.

60. Stanley Wright to JBR, January 28, 1970, box 9, folder 9, JBR Papers.

61. The inclusion criteria were chronological age of three to six years at study onset, IQ (per Stanford-Binet Test) between fifty and eighty-four, lower socioeconomic class, one or both parents diagnosed as "mentally subnormal," at least one sibling diagnosed as "mentally subnormal," and lack of gross neurological findings (Robert B. Kugel and Mabel Parsons, *Children of Deprivation: Changing the Course of Familial Mental Retardation* [Washington, D.C.: U.S. Department of Health, Education, and Welfare, Welfare Administration, Children's Bureau, 1967], 14).

62. Ibid., i.

63. This intervention resembles the enrichment programs developed in the early 1960s that later served as models for Project Head Start. See, for example, Bettye M. Caldwell and Julius B. Richmond, "Programmed Day Care for the Very Young Child: A Preliminary Report," *Journal of Marriage and Family* 26, no. 4 (1964): 481–88.

64. Kugel and Parsons, *Children of Deprivation*, 24.

65. Ibid., 24–25.

66. Ibid., 48.

67. Ibid., 57.

68. Mabel Parsons, "A Home Economist in Service to Families with Mental Retardation," *Children* 7, no. 5 (1960): 188.

69. Robert Kugel, "The Forgotten Retarded: In Residential Facilities, in Poverty," paper presented at the Joint Membership Meeting of the Minneapolis and St. Paul Associations for Retarded Children, April 24, 1968, 8, http://www.mnddc.state.mn.us /parallels2/pdf/index.html.

70. Howard Garber, *The Milwaukee Project: Preventing Mental Retardation in Children at Risk* (Washington, D.C.: American Association on Mental Retardation, 1988), 30–31.

71. Richard J. Herrnstein and Charles Murray, *The Bell Curve: Intelligence and Class Structure in American Life* (New York: Free Press, 1994), 408.

72. Kenneth A. Kavale and Mark P. Mostert, *The Positive Side of Special Education: Minimizing Its Fads, Fancies, and Follies* (Lanham, Md.: Rowman and Littlefield, 2004), 24.

73. Seth S. King, "Test Finds I.Q.'s Can Be Lifted for Children of Retarded," *New York Times*, July 17, 1972; Stephen P. Strickland, "Can Slum Children Learn?," in *The Fallacy of IQ*, ed. Carl Senna (New York: Third Press, 1973), 150–59.

74. Ellis B. Page, "Miracle in Milwaukee: Raising the IQ," *Educational Researcher* 1, no. 10 (1972): 8.

75. Kavale and Mostert, *Positive Side*, 25; Robert Sommer and Barbara A. Sommer, "Mystery in Milwaukee: Early Intervention, IQ, and Psychology Textbooks," *American Psychologist* 38, no. 9 (1983): 983.

76. Arthur Jensen, "Raising IQ without Increasing G?: A Review of the Milwaukee Project: Preventing Mental Retardation in Children at Risk," *Developmental Review* 9, no. 3 (1989): 237.

77. Richard Heber and Howard Garber, "An Experiment in the Prevention of Cultural-Familial Mental Retardation," 7, paper presented at the Second Congress of the International Association for the Scientific Study of Mental Deficiency, Warsaw, Poland, August 25–September 2, 1970.

78. Ibid., 6.

79. Howard Garber and Richard Heber, *The Milwaukee Project: Early Intervention as a Technique to Prevent Mental Retardation* (Storrs: University of Connecticut, National Leadership Institute, 1973), 11.

80. Garber, *The Milwaukee Project: Preventing Mental Retardation in Children at Risk*, 49–67. Garber's publication, which appeared nearly two decades after the intervention had begun and after Heber's death, provides much-needed detail on the program. Yet because of this program's troubled history and the belated publication date, I did not examine its reliance on theories of deprivation but instead focused only on publications from the 1960s.

81. Jensen, "Raising IQ," 245.

82. Reginald Lourie and Dorothy Huntington, "Proposal for a Program to Prevent Culturally Determined Intellectual Retardation and Personal Dysfunction," June 1968, 8, box 1257, folder 4, G&LBM Papers; Allen E. Marans, Dale R. Meers, and Dorothy S. Huntington, "The Children's Hospital in Washington, D.C.," in *Early Child Care: The New Perspectives*, ed. Caroline A. Chandler, Reginald S. Lourie, and Anne D. Peters (New York: Atherton, 1968), 287–301.

83. Secretary's Committee on Mental Retardation, *Mental Retardation Grants, Fiscal Year 1966* (Washington, D.C.: U.S. Department of Health, Education and Welfare,

1966), http://www.mnddc.org/dd_act/documents/construction/66–MRG-HEW .pdf.

84. For example, in 1964, the *Washington Post* reported a $216,000 NIMH grant to Lourie and Allen E. Marans for an early intervention program targeting culturally deprived infants that was remarkably similar to the Lourie and Huntington project ("Unloved Infants to Get Vital Break," *Washington Post*, December 20, 1964). Beginning in 1968, Lourie and a junior colleague, Dale R. Meers, conducted a study on "Culturally Determined Retardation: Clinical Explorations of Variability and Etiology" that was supported by private philanthropic organizations as well as by the Baltimore Psychoanalytic Society. Meers described this project as a continuation of the earlier NIMH-funded project. Lourie and Meers's project yielded numerous publications but did not describe the actual intervention funded by Lourie and Huntington's NIMH grant. See "News and Proceedings of Affiliate Societies and Institutes," *Bulletin of the American Psychoanalytic Association* 24 (1968): 854–67; Dale R. Meers, "Contributions of a Ghetto Culture to Symptom Formation—Psychoanalytic Studies of Ego Anomalies in Childhood," *Psychoanalytic Study of the Child* 25 (1970): 209–30; Dale R. Meers, "Psychoanalytic Research and Intellectual Functioning of Ghetto-Reared, Black Children," *Psychoanalytic Study of the Child* 28 (1973): 395–417; Dale R. Meers, "Traumatic and Cultural Distortions of Psychoneurotic Symptoms in a Black Ghetto," *Annual of Psychoanalysis* 2 (1974): 368–86.

85. Lourie and Huntington, "Proposal for a Program," i.

86. Ibid., 8.

87. Ibid., 7.

88. Ibid., i, 4.

89. Ibid., 4.

90. Ibid., 5.

91. Ibid., ii.

92. The proposal cites the National Committee on Civil Disorder's laudatory description of the benefits of Project Head Start and other early intervention programs to demonstrate the importance of early childhood enrichment (ibid.).

93. A detailed account of this lawsuit appears in Raymond Wolters, *The Burden of Brown: Thirty Years of School Desegregation* (Knoxville: University of Tennessee Press, 1984), 9–52. Wolters is a longtime critic of *Brown v. Board of Education* who has consistently argued for the plausibility of a genetic intellectual inferiority of African Americans. His work has been criticized for scholarly shortcomings or misinterpretations that have consistently advanced his political bias. See also Raymond Wolters, *Race and Education, 1954–2007* (Columbia: University of Missouri Press, 2009), x; David J. Garrow, "Segregation's Legacy," *Reviews in American History* 13, no. 3 (1985): 428–32.

94. Richard L. Lyons and Eve Edstrom, "Integration Called Miracle of Social Adjustment Here," *Washington Post*, February 11, 1957; Gerald Grant, "Hansen and Aides Review Eight Years of Desegregation in Schools of District," *Washington Post*, November 18, 1962; "'Integrated' Primers Get Hansen Nod," *Washington Post*, December 26, 1963.

95. Erwin Knoll, "District School Rolls Declared 73.8% Negro," *Washington Post*, September 5, 1958; "Big City Answers," *Time*, July 9, 1965; Wolters, *Burden of Brown*, 18–23.

96. The case had originally alleged that because the District's school board members

were appointed directly by district court judges, the case could not be heard by any district court judge (Wolters, *Burden of Brown*, 31–33; Thomas W. Lippman, "Wright Edict Upheld on All Major Points," *Washington Post*, January 22, 1969).

97. See, for example, "Impact Varies in Ban on Track System," *Washington Post*, December 16, 1967.

98. William Raspberry, "Ban on Track System Deals Blow at Classes for Retarded Children," *Washington Post*, September 15, 1967.

99. "Impact Varies in Ban on Track System," *Washington Post*, December 16, 1967.

100. Ben A. Franklin, "School Head Quits in Washington Rift over Racial Policy," *New York Times*, July 4, 1967; Susan Jacoby, "The Superintendent Simply Stood Still," *Washington Post*, July 9, 1967; Ben A. Franklin, "Hansen Is Seeking to Appeal Order," *New York Times*, July 18, 1967.

101. Osgood, *History of Inclusion*, 80–84; Harry and Klingner, *Why Are So Many Minority Students*, 2; Blanchett, Mumford, and Beachum, "Urban School Failure," 74.

102. Lloyd Dunn, "Special Education for the Mildly Retarded—Is Much of It Justifiable?," *Exceptional Children* 35, no. 1 (1965): 6.

103. Ibid., 7.

104. In 1987, Dunn published a controversial monograph that suggested that genetic factors might be involved in Latino-white differences in intelligence. Widely criticized, Dunn ultimately published an apology, though it did little to improve his image in the eyes of antiracist educators (Richard Valencia and Lisa Suzuki, *Intelligence Testing and Minority Students* [Thousand Oaks, Calif.: Sage, 2001], 169–72; Richard Valencia, *Dismantling Contemporary Deficit Thinking: Educational Thought and Practice* [New York: Routledge, 2010], 47–48).

105. President's Committee on Mental Retardation, *The Six-Hour Retarded Child: A Report on a Conference on Problems of Education in Children in the Inner City* (Washington, D.C.: U.S. Office of Education, 1969), 3.

106. The seven recommendations were (1) provide early childhood stimulation, education, and evaluation as part of the continuum of public education; (2) conduct a study of histories of successful inner-city families who have learned to cope effectively with their environment; (3) restructure the education of teachers, administrators, counselors and retrain those now in the field; (4) reexamine the present system of intelligence testing and classification; (5) commit substantial additional funding for research and development in educational improvement for disadvantaged children and youth; (6) thoroughly delineate what constitutes accountability, allocate sufficient funds to carry out the responsibility entailed, and hold schools accountable for providing quality education for all children; and (7) involve parents, citizens and citizen groups, students, and general and special educators in the total educational effort (ibid., 8).

107. Wilson C. Riles, "Educating Inner City Children: Challenges and Opportunities," paper presented at the President's Committee on Mental Retardation's Conference on Problems of Education of Children in the Inner City, Warrenton, Virginia, August 10–12, 1969, in *Disadvantaged Child*, vol. 3, *Compensatory Education: A National Debate*, ed. Jerome Hellmuth (New York: Bruner/Mazel, 1970), 273.

108. *Larry P. v. Riles*, No. C-71 2270, 343 F. Supp. 1306, 1972, U.S. Dist. LEXIS 13149,

June 20, 1972; Asa G. Hilliard III, "IQ and the Courts: *Larry P. v. Wilson Riles* and *PASE v. Hannon*," in *African American Psychology: Theory, Research, and Practice*, ed. A. Kathleen Hoard Burlew, W. Curtis Banks, Harriette Pipes McAdoo, and Daudi Ajani ya Azibo (Newbury Park, Calif.: Sage, 1992), 199–218; Osgood, *History of Inclusion*, 104; Scott Graves and Angela Mitchell, "Is the Moratorium Over?: African American Psychology Professionals' Views on Intelligence Testing in Response to Changes to Federal Policy," *Journal of Black Psychology* 37, no. 4 (1965): 407–25.

109. Charles R. Tremper, "Organized Psychology's Efforts to Influence Judicial Policy-Making," *American Psychologist* 42, no. 5 (1987): 497–98.

110. *Larry P. v. Riles*, No. C-71-2270 RFP, 495 F. Supp. 926, October 16, 1979.

111. *Larry P. v. Riles*. No 80-4027, 793 F.2d 969; 1984 U.S. App., LEXIS 26195, January 23, 1984.

112. "Suit Challenges Score," *Los Angeles Times*, November 23, 1977.

113. Joel Dreyfuss, "Wilson Riles Speaks Out," *Black Enterprise* 8, no. 12 (1978): 35–38; Elaine Woo, "Wilson Riles, First Black Elected to State Office, Dies," *Los Angeles Times*, April 3, 1999.

114. See, for example, "California's New Education Boss," *Ebony*, May 1971, 54–56; "California Children to Start School at Age Four," *Jet*, April 5, 1973; "The 100 Most Influential Black Americans," *Ebony*, May 1974, 92.

115. Wilson C. Riles, "'No Adversary Situations': Public School Education in California and Wilson C. Riles, Superintendent of Public Instruction, 1970–1982," interview by Sarah Sharp, 1981–82, Bancroft Library, University of California, Berkeley; "Educator Named Spingarn Medalist," *Crisis*, June–July 1973, 211.

116. According to literature from the early to mid-1960s, 85 percent of those labeled "mentally retarded" were categorized as "mild" (Harvey A. Stevens, "Overview," in *Mental Retardation*, ed. Stevens and Heber, 5).

117. James Clements and Sue Warren, "History of the Classification of Mental Retardation," June 1978, Herbert J. Grossman, M.D., Collection, box 1, folder 20, Archives and Special Collections, Department of the Library, College of Staten Island, City University of New York, Staten Island.

118. Donovan and Cross, *Minority Students*, 45–47.

119. U.S. Congress, *Amendment to the Individuals with Disabilities Education Act*, January 7, 1997, Section 618. Since 2000, Indicator 9 of Section 300.600(a)(2) of IDEA has required that states monitor and avoid disproportionate representation of racial or ethnic groups in special education as a result of inappropriate identification policies.

120. Henry Leland, "Poverty and Mental Retardation," *Clinical Child Psychology Newsletter* 9, no. 2 (1970): 4.

121. Michael B. Katz, a longtime poverty scholar and historian, has described the term "undeserving poor" as an "enduring attempt to classify poor people by merit." This and related terms enable a debate over who is, by virtue of behavior and character, entitled to receive what are perceived as resources belonging to others (*The Undeserving Poor: From the War on Poverty to the War on Welfare* [New York: Pantheon, 1989], 9–15).

122. Dunn, "Special Education," 6.

123. Donovan and Cross, *Minority Students*, 2; Harry and Klingner, *Why Are So Many Minority Students*, 2–3; Ferri and Connor, "Tools of Exclusion," 458.

124. *Intellectual Disability: Definition, Classification, and Systems of Supports* (Washington, D.C.: American Association on Intellectual and Developmental Disabilities, 2010), 59–60.

CHAPTER FIVE

1. Martin Gansberg, "37 Who Saw Murder Didn't Call the Police," *New York Times*, March 27, 1964.

2. Stanley Milgram and Paul Hollander, "The Murder They Heard," *The Nation*, June 15, 1964, 602–4; Stanley Milgram, "The Experience of Living in Cities," *Science* 167, no. 3924 (1970): 1461–68; Rachel Manning, Mark Levine, and Alan Collins, "The Kitty Genovese Murder and the Social Psychology of Helping: The Parable of the 38 Witnesses," *American Psychologist* 62, no. 6 (2007): 555–62. A number of behavioral science experts speculated on this supposed urban detachment in the *New York Times* (Charles Mour, "Apathy Is Puzzle in Queens Killing," *New York Times*, March 28, 1964).

3. J. H. Bradbury, "Walden Three: New Environmentalism, Urban Design, and Planning in the Nineteen Sixties," *Antipode* 8, no. 3 (1976): 17–28.

4. Kevin Kruse, *White Flight: Atlanta and the Making of Modern Conservatism* (Princeton: Princeton University Press, 2005).

5. Eric Avila, *Popular Culture in the Age of White Flight: Fear and Fantasy in Suburban Los Angeles* (Berkeley: University of California Press, 2004), 70–74.

6. Thomas Sugrue, *The Origins of the Urban Crisis: Race and Inequality in Postwar Detroit* (Princeton: Princeton University Press, 1996), 8–9.

7. This game was first distributed as a pullout in the August 1968 issue of *Psychology Today* and was later available for separate purchase. See David Popoff, "The Cities Game," *Psychology Today* 2, no. 3 (1968): 38–40.

8. Mark H. Lytle, *The Gentle Subversive: Rachel Carson, Silent Spring, and the Rise of the Environmental Movement* (New York: Oxford University Press, 2007).

9. Group for the Advancement of Psychiatry, *Urban America and the Planning of Mental Health Services* (New York: GAP, 1964).

10. Ibid., 411–14.

11. Joachim F. Wohlwill, "The Emerging Discipline of Environmental Psychology," *American Psychologist* 25, no. 4 (1970): 303–12; Harold Proshansky, William Ittelson, and Leanne Rivlin, eds., *Environmental Psychology: Man and His Physical Setting* (New York: Holt, Rinehart, and Winston, 1970).

12. Paul Leyhausen, "The Communal Organization of Solitary Mammals," in *Environmental Psychology*, ed. Proshansky, Ittelson, and Rivlin, 183.

13. *Report of the National Advisory Commission on Civil Disorders* (New York: Bantam, 1968), 5–7; Joseph Boskin, *Urban Racial Violence in the Twentieth Century*, 2nd ed. (Beverly Hills, Calif.: Glencoe, 1976), 101–42; Robert M. Fogelson, *Violence as Protest: A Study of Riots and Ghettos* (Garden City, N.Y.: Doubleday, 1971), 1–52.

14. Kenneth Neubeck and Noel Cazenave, *Welfare Racism: Playing the Race Card against America's Poor* (New York: Routledge, 2001), 116–24.

15. Edmund Ramsen and Jon Adams, "Escaping the Laboratory: The Rodent Experi-

ments of John B. Calhoun and Their Cultural Influence," *Journal of Social History* 42, no. 3 (2009): 761–92.

16. Leonard Duhl, ed. *The Urban Condition: People and Policy in the Metropolis* (1963; New York: Simon and Schuster, 1969), xiii; Ramsen and Adams, "Escaping the Laboratory," 767; Joe Flower, "Building Healthier Cities: A Conversation with Leonard J. Duhl," *Healthcare Forum Journal* 36, no. 3 (1993): 48–54, 75.

17. Omer R. Galle, Walter R. Gove, and J. Miller McPherson, "Population Density and Pathology: What Are the Relations for Man?," *Science* 176, no. 4030 (1972): 24.

18. René Dubos, "We Can't Buy Our Way Out," *Psychology Today* 3, no. 10 (1970): 20–22, 86–87, René Dubos, "Man Overadapting," *Psychology Today* 4, no. 9 (1971): 50–53.

19. Carol L. Moberg, *René Dubos: Friend of the Good Earth* (Washington, D.C.: ASM Press, 2005), 147–50.

20. René Dubos, *Man Adapting* (New Haven: Yale University Press, 1965), xxi, 25.

21. Ibid., 26.

22. René Dubos, "The Crisis of Man in His Environment," in *Human Identity in the Urban Environment*, ed. Gwen Bell and Jacqueline Tyrwhitt (Harmondsworth: Penguin, 1972), 183–84 (first published in *Proceedings of the Symposium on Human Ecology* [Washington, D.C.: U.S. Public Health Service, 1968]).

23. Everett M. Rogers, "The Extensions of Men: The Correspondence of Marshall McLuhan and Edward T. Hall," *Mass Communication and Society* 3, no. 1 (2000): 117–35.

24. Edward T. Hall, "The Silent Language in Overseas Business," *Harvard Business Review*, May 1960, 87–96; Edward T. Hall and Mildred Hall, "The Sounds of Silence," *Playboy*, June 1971, 139–40, 204, 206.

25. Edward T. Hall, *The Hidden Dimension* (New York: Anchor, 1966), 1.

26. Ibid., 177, 171.

27. Ibid., 168.

28. Parr was a frequent speaker to nonspecialized audiences on popular scientific topics and was often mentioned in the *New York Times* and other newspapers and magazines. See, for example, "Science: Weather Control?," *Time*, July 5, 1943; "Making 'Natural History Live,'" *New York Times*, April 5, 1959.

29. Albert E. Parr, "City and Psyche," *Yale Review* 55 (1965): 80–81.

30. Albert E. Parr, "Psychological Aspects of Urbanology," *Social Issues* 22, no. 4 (1966): 42.

31. James E. Montgomery, "Impact of Housing Patterns on Marital Interaction," *Family Coordinator* 19, no. 3 (1970): 271.

32. Paul Lemkau, "A Psychiatrist's View of Housing," in *Proceedings: Seventh Conference for the Improvement of the Teaching of Housing in Home Economics, October 30–November 2, 1963*, 10, series 3, box 2, folder 4, American Association of Housing Educators Records, Cushing Memorial Library, Texas A&M University, College Station.

33. Betty Friedan, *The Feminine Mystique* (New York: Norton, 1963).

34. Ibid., 393–428; Kirsten Fermaglich, *American Dreams and Nazi Nightmares: Early Holocaust Consciousness and Liberal America, 1957–1965* (Waltham, Mass.: Brandeis University Press; Hanover, N.H.: University Press of New England, 2006), 58–82; Daniel Horowitz, *Betty Friedan and the Making of The Feminine Mystique: The American Left,*

the Cold War, and Modern Feminism (Amherst: University of Massachusetts Press, 1998).

35. James Howard Kunstler, *Home from Nowhere: Remaking Our Everyday World for the Twenty-First Century* (New York: Simon and Schuster, 1996); Nicholas Bloom, *Suburban Alchemy: 1960s New Towns and the Transformation of the American Dream* (Columbus: Ohio State University Press, 2001), 208–9; Lizabeth Cohen, *A Consumers' Republic: The Politics of Mass Consumption in Postwar America* (New York: Knopf, 2003), 193–256.

36. Leonard Duhl, "Looking Backwards: A Personal Look at Community Mental Health," *Journal of Primary Prevention* 15, no. 1 (1994): 31–43; Flower, "Building Healthier Cities," 48–52.

37. On Dubos's role in the development of ekistics and his influence on Doxiadis, see Ellen Shoskes and Sy Adler, "Planning for Healthy People/Healthy Places: Lessons from Mid-Twentieth Century Global Discourse," *Planning Perspectives* 24, no. 2 (2009): 197–217.

38. "Biographical Sketches," *Social Issues* 22, no. 4 (1966): 137–40.

39. Robert W. Kates, "Stimulus and Symbol: The View from the Bridge," *Social Issues* 22, no. 4 (1966): 23.

40. Robert Sommer, "Man's Proximate Environment," *Social Issues* 22, no. 4 (1966): 59.

41. Wohlwill, "Emerging Discipline," 305, 307–8, 310. Harry Heft, Wohlwill's former student, refers to this publication as a landmark that introduced the field of environmental psychology to many readers ("Joachim F. Wohlwill (1928–1987): His Contributions to the Emerging Discipline of Environmental Psychology," *Environment and Behavior* 20 [1988]: 260).

42. Harold Searles, *The Nonhuman Environment in Normal Development and in Schizophrenia* (New York: International Universities Press, 1960), 5.

43. Ibid., 49–51.

44. Ibid., 166.

45. In 1963, Searles published an article in the *International Journal of Psycho-Analysis* examining the interrelations between sensory deprivation and schizophrenia. An interaction with a patient had led him to understand the "previously unsuspected intensity of sensory deprivation in the subjective experience of various other schizophrenic patients" ("The Place of Neutral Therapist-Responses in Psychotherapy with the Schizophrenic Patient," *International Journal of Psycho-Analysis* 44 [1963]: 42).

46. Stuart C. Miller, "Ego-Autonomy in Sensory Deprivation, Isolation, and Stress," *International Journal of Psycho-Analysis* 43 (1962): 6. See also Lawrence S. Kubie, "Theoretical Aspects of Sensory Deprivation," in *Sensory Deprivation: A Symposium Held at Harvard Medical School*, ed. Philip Solomon, Philip E. Kubzansky, P. Herbert Leiderman Jr., Jack H. Mendelson, Richard Trumbull, and Donald Wexler (Cambridge: Harvard University Press, 1961), 208–20.

47. John E. S. Lawrence, "Science and Sentiment: Overview of Research on Crowding and Human Behavior," *Psychological Bulletin* 81, no. 10 (1974): 712–20.

48. Robert E. Mitchell, "Some Social Implications of High Density Housing," *American Sociological Review* 36, no. 1 (1971): 19–20.

49. Alvin Schorr, *Slums and Social Insecurity* (Washington, D.C.: U.S. Department of Health Education and Welfare, 1963), 1–2.

50. Ibid., 18.

51. Joseph Boskin, "The Revolt of the Urban Ghettos, 1964–1967," *Annals of the American Academy of Political and Social Science* 382 (1969): 1–14; Stanley Lieberson and Arnold R. Silverman, "The Precipitants and Underlying Conditions of Race Riots," *American Sociological Review* 30, no. 6 (1965): 887–98; Walter Rucker and James Upton, eds., *Encyclopedia of American Race Riots* (Westport, Conn.: Greenwood, 2007), 478–79.

52. Rucker and Upton, *Encyclopedia of American Race Riots*, 507, 511.

53. Robert M. Fogelson, "White on Black: A Critique of the McCone Commission Report on the Los Angeles Riots," *Political Science Quarterly* 82, no. 3 (1967): 337–67; David O. Sears and John B. McConahay, "Participation in the Los Angeles Riot," *Social Problems* 17, no. 1 (1969): 15–16; Lindsey Lupo, *Flak-Catchers: One Hundred Years of Riot Commission Politics in America* (Lanham, Md.: Lexington, 2011), 93–122.

54. Ellen Herman, *The Romance of American Psychology: Political Culture in the Age of Experts* (Berkeley: University of California Press, 1995), 232.

55. Sugrue, *Origins of the Urban Crisis*, 259–68; Amy Maria Kenyon, *Dreaming Suburbia: Detroit and the Production of Postwar Space and Culture* (Detroit: Wayne State University Press, 2004), 9–15.

56. "Remarks of the President upon Issuing an Executive Order Establishing a National Advisory Commission on Civil Disorders," July 29, 1967, in *Report of the National Advisory Commission*, 536–37; Herman, *Romance of American Psychology*, 210. For an in-depth analysis of the Kerner Commission's deliberations, see Michael Lipsky and David J. Olson, *Commission Politics: The Processing of Racial Crisis in America* (New Brunswick, N.J.: Transaction, 1977), 107–230.

57. Herman, *Romance of American Psychology*, 216–18; Robert Shellow, "Social Scientists and Social Action from within the Establishment," *Journal of Social Issues* 26, no. 1 (1970): 208; Lupo, *Flak Catchers*, 134–35.

58. Herman, *Romance of American Psychology*, 217.

59. Charles Pinderhughes, "Pathogenic Social Structure: A Prime Target for Preventative Psychiatric Intervention," *Journal of the National Medical Association* 58, no. 6 (1966): 424.

60. Charles Pinderhughes and Herbert Levin, "Psychology of Adolescents in a Peaceful Protest and in an Urban Riot," November 6, 1967, reel 27, 511–49, KC Records.

61. "Psychiatry: Understanding Militancy," *Time*, May 24, 1968; Pinderhughes, "Pathogenic Social Structure," 428; Jane Brody, "Doctor Analyzes Black Power Idea," *New York Times*, May 16, 1968.

62. Pinderhughes, "Pathogenic Social Structure," 427.

63. Ibid., 426.

64. Pinderhughes and Levin, "Psychology of Adolescents," 533.

65. Kevin Mumford, "Harvesting the Crisis: The Newark Uprising, the Kerner Commission, and Writing on Riots," in *African American Urban History since World War II*, ed. Kenneth Kusmer and Joe W. Trotter (Chicago: University of Chicago Press, 2009), 209–10.

66. Alondra Nelson, *Body and Soul: The Black Panther Party and the Fight against Medical Discrimination* (Minneapolis: University of Minnesota Press, 2011), 153–68; Michael Staub, *Madness Is Civilization: When the Diagnosis Was Social, 1948–1980* (Chicago: University of Chicago Press, 2011), 124–26.

67. Jonathan Metzl, *The Protest Psychosis: How Schizophrenia Became a Black Disease* (Boston: Beacon, 2010), 95–128.

68. Vernon Mark, William Sweet, and Frank Ervin, "Role of Brain Disease in Riots and Urban Violence," *Journal of the American Medical Association* 201, no. 11 (1967): 895.

69. Nelson, *Body and Soul*, 153–68; Staub, *Madness Is Civilization*, 125.

70. The popular press printed frequent updates regarding the Kerner Commission's progress. See, for example, Donald Janson, "Kerner Pledges Thorough Study of Urban Rioting," *New York Times*, July 29, 1967; "Text of Summary of Report by National Advisory Commission on Civil Disorders," *New York Times*, March 1, 1968; "Kerner Is Unsure on Riots Meeting," *New York Times*, April 12, 1968.

71. *Report of the National Advisory Commission.*

72. Clarence W. Klassen to Christopher Vlahoplus, August 4, 1967, reel 13, 7801, KC Records; Michael Halberstam to Joseph Califano, July 28, 1967, reel 13, 786, KC Records; Jacquelyne Jackson to Lyndon Johnson, July 28, 1967, reel 13, 642, KC Records.

73. Herman, *Romance of American Psychology*, 224.

74. Ibid., 237; Peter Lupsha, "On Theories of Urban Violence," *Urban Affairs Quarterly* 4, no. 3 (1969): 273–96. Lipsky and Olson provide a scathing critique of attempts to depoliticize and delegitimize insurgent groups and their goals (*Commission Politics*, 443–59). A concrete illustration of these attempts to depoliticize riots can be seen in an item in the *Science News-Letter* that sported an unambiguous subtitle: "Extreme poverty and social deprivation, rather than civil rights issues, lead to resentments, mental imbalance and violence" (Faye Marley, "Poverty Causes Violence," *Science News-Letter*, August 22, 1964, 114).

75. *Report of the National Advisory Commission*, 123, 325; William Griffitt and Russell Veitch, "Hot and Crowded: Influences of Population Density and Temperature on Interpersonal Affective Behavior," *Journal of Personality and Social Psychology* 17, no. 1 (1971): 93.

76. For a history of the concept of relative deprivation, see Francine Tougas and Ann M. Beaton, "Personal Relative Deprivation: A Look at the Grievous Consequences of Grievance," *Social and Personality Psychology Compass* 2, no. 4 (2008): 1753–66.

77. Siddharth Chadra and Angela Williams Foster, "The 'Revolution of Rising Expectations,' Relative Deprivation, and the Urban Social Disorders of the 1960s: Evidence from State-Level Data," *Social Science History* 29, no. 2 (2005): 299–332; Don R. Bowen, Elinor R. Bowen, Sheldon R. Gawiser, and Louis H. Masotti, "Deprivation, Mobility, and Orientation toward Protest of the Urban Poor," *American Behavioral Scientist* 11, no. 4 (1968): 20–24; Thomas J. Crawford and Murray Naditch, "Relative Deprivation, Powerlessness, and Militancy: The Psychology of Social Protest," *Psychiatry* 33, no. 2 (1970): 208–23.

78. Kenneth B. Clark, statement, September 13, 1967, reel 3, 1263, KC Records; John Gardner, statement, August 1, 1967, reel 1, 86–87, KC Records; Herman, *Romance of American Psychology*, 220.

79. Andreas Hess, *Concepts of Social Stratification: European and American Models* (New York: Palgrave, 2001), 161–67; Seymour Martin Lipset, "Comments on the Problems of Urban Ghettos and Issues of Public Order," discussion paper for the RAND Urban Programs Workshop, December 1967–January 1968, reel 22, 281, KC Records (published as Seymour M. Lipset, "The Problems of Urban Ghettos and the Issues of Public Order," in *Thinking about Cities: New Perspectives on Urban Problems*, ed. Anthony Pascal [Belmont, Calif.: Dickenson, 1970], 140–52).

80. Ursula Dibble, "Socially Shared Deprivation, Participation in Non-Violent Protest, and the Approval of Violence" (Ph.D. diss., University of Connecticut, 1978); Susan Olzak and Suzanne Shanahan, "Deprivation and Race Riots: An Extension of Spilerman's Analysis," *Social Forces* 74, no. 3 (1996): 931–61; Stephen G. Brush, "Dynamics of Theory Change in the Social Sciences: Relative Deprivation and Collective Violence," *Journal of Conflict Resolution* 40, no. 4 (1996): 523–45.

81. John Gardner, statement, reel 1, 371, KC Records; Louis H. Masotti, "Preface," *American Behavioral Scientist* 2, no. 4 (1968): 1; Herman, *Romance of American Psychology*, 218.

82. "Toward an Understanding of Mass Violence: Contributions from the Behavioral Sciences," NIMH confidential report, August 1967, reel 15, 372, KC Records.

83. Ibid., 4.

84. Martin Luther King Jr., statement, October 23, 1967, reel 4, 963, KC Records.

85. Ibid., 958.

86. Martin Luther King Jr., *Why We Can't Wait* (New York: Harper and Row, 1964), 152. In his statement before the Kerner Commission, King argued that the "bill of rights for the disadvantaged" would apply to whites as well as blacks (reel 4, 961, KC Records).

87. King, *Why We Can't Wait*, 153, 141.

88. Martin Luther King Jr., Nobel lecture, December 11, 1964, http://www.nobel prize.org/nobel_prizes/peace/laureates/1964/king-lecture.html.

89. King made similar suggestions in a 1965 interview for *Playboy* magazine (Alex Haley, "Interview with Martin Luther King," *Playboy*, January 1965, 70–71).

90. Throughout his career, King appropriated material, often verbatim, into his sermons, writings, and academic work, frequently without the customary documentation. When this practice was uncovered in the late 1980s, considerable controversy erupted regarding King's legacy and academic credentials. A committee of scholars at Boston University, which had granted King his doctorate, concluded that King had plagiarized parts of his dissertation, leading to the decision to append a note to the university's copy of the work. While King's misappropriation of material in his academic work has been universally criticized, his tendency to borrow and synthesize from a wide range of sources in his sermons has been tied to the oral tradition of black folk preachers. See David Thelen, "Becoming Martin Luther King, Jr.: An Introduction," *Journal of American History* 78, no. 1 (1991): 11–22; Clayborne Carson, Peter Holloran, Ralph E. Luker, and Penny Russell, "Martin Luther King, Jr., as Scholar: A Reexamination of His Theological Writings," *Journal of American History* 78, no. 1 (1991): 93–105; Keith D. Miller, "Martin Luther King, Jr., and the Black Folk Pulpit," *Journal of American History* 78, no. 1 (1991): 120–23; "Boston U. Panel Finds Plagiarism by Dr. King," *New York Times*, October 11, 1991; Keith D. Miller, *Voice of Deliverance: The Language of Martin Luther King, Jr., and Its Sources* (New York: Free Press, 1992).

91. In his work on the "damage imagery" of the African American psyche, historian Daryl M. Scott examines how black intellectuals linked this imagery to demands for compensatory programs targeting blacks (*Contempt and Pity: Social Policy and the Image of the Damaged Black Psyche, 1880–1996* [Chapel Hill: University of North Carolina Press, 1997], 138, 148–50).

92. Ibid., 149; Karen Ferguson, "Organizing the Ghetto: The Ford Foundation, CORE, and White Power in the Black Power Era," *Journal of Urban History* 34, no. 1 (2007): 67–99.

93. Willie E. Thompson to William B. Spong, August 21, 1967, reel 14, 13, KC Records.

94. Herman, *Romance of American Psychology*, 219–22; Kevin Mumford, "Untangling Pathology: The Moynihan Report and Homosexual Damage, 1965–1975," *Journal of Policy History* 24, no. 1 (2012): 53–73.

95. Lupo, *Flak Catchers*, 137–40; John Gardner, statement, reel 1, 95–96, KC Records.

96. Clarice U. Heckert to Kerner Commission, August 25, 1967, reel 13, 704, KC Records.

97. Elliot Liebow, *Tally's Corner: A Study of Negro Streetcorner Men* (Boston: Little, Brown, 1967). See also James D. Montgomery, "Revisiting Tally's Corner: Mainstream Norms, Cognitive Dissonance, and Underclass Behavior," *Rationality and Society* 6 (October 1994): 462–88; Herman, *Romance of American Psychology*, 221–22; Mitchell Duneier, "On the Legacy of Elliot Liebow and Carol Stack: Context-Driven Fieldwork and the Need for Continuous Ethnography," *Focus* 25, no. 1 (2007): 33–38.

98. Commission Meeting Transcripts, November 9, 1967, reel 5, 3712, 3715, KC Records.

99. Commission Meeting Transcripts, November 9, 1967, reel 5, 3719, 3750, KC Records.

100. Commission Meeting Transcripts, November 9, 1967, reel 5, 3729, 3736, KC Records. Analyses and interpretations of the locus of control among the poor (internal versus external control) and the attempt to empower populations seen to be powerless or motivate them to develop more "internal control" provided the basis for different governmental interventions during the War on Poverty. See Karen Baistow, "Problems of Powerlessness: Psychological Explanations of Social Inequality and Civil Unrest in Post-War America," *History of the Human Sciences* 13, no. 3 (2000): 95–116.

101. Commission Meeting Transcripts, November 9, 1967, reel 5, 3775, KC Records.

102. Ibid., 3572.

103. Ibid., 3574.

104. For a fuller discussion of the interrelations among maternal employment, race, and welfare eligibility, see Jill Quadagno, *The Color of Welfare: How Racism Undermined the War on Poverty* (Oxford: Oxford University Press, 1994).

105. Commission Meeting Transcripts, November 9, 1967, reel 5, 3757, KC Records.

106. Duhl, "Looking Back," 40.

107. Matthew Dumont, *The Absurd Healer: Perspective of a Community Psychiatrist* (New York: Science House, 1968).

108. Ibid., 54–55.

109. Ibid., 66.

110. Ibid., 67.

111. Ibid., 68–71.

112. Ibid., 50–51.

113. Ibid., 75–77.

114. Ibid., 80.

115. Lupo, *Flak Catchers*, 139–40.

116. Mumford, "Harvesting the Crisis," 209.

117. *Report of the National Advisory Commission*, 2. On this point, see Herman, *Romance of American Psychology*, 232.

118. *Report of the National Advisory Commission*, 10–11.

119. Ibid., 226, 244, 258–59.

120. Ibid., 22–23.

121. Ibid., 395, 403–5.

122. Ibid., 262.

123. Ibid., 446.

124. Ibid., 449.

125. Ibid., 427.

126. Lupo, *Flak Catchers*, 147–49.

127. Herman, *Romance of American Psychology*, 243–46; Claire Jean Kim, "Clinton's Race Initiative: Recasting the American Dilemma," *Polity* 33, no. 2 (2000): 185.

128. Richard L. Meier, "Violence: The Last Urban Epidemic," *American Behavioral Scientist* 11, no. 4 (1968): 35.

CONCLUSION

1. Sarah Huisenga, "Newt Gingrich: Poor Kids Don't Work 'Unless It's Illegal,'" December 1, 2011, http://www.cbsnews.com/8301–503544_162–57335118–503544/newt-gingrich-poor-kids-dont-work-unless-its-illegal/; Karen Tumulty, "Gingrich Urges Students to Get Part-Time Jobs," *Washington Post*, January 28, 2012.

2. Maris A. Vinovskis, *The Birth of Head Start: Preschool Education Policies in the Kennedy and Johnson Administrations* (Chicago: University of Chicago Press, 2005), 76–89, 149–52.

3. Society for Research in Child Development, "Award History," http://www.srcd .org/index.php?option=com_content&task=view&id=153&Itemid=0.

4. Mieke Bal, *Travelling Concepts in the Humanities: A Rough Guide* (Toronto: University of Toronto Press, 2002).

5. Tom Levin, "A Social Action Analysis of Head Start," *American Journal of Public Health and the Nation's Health* 57, no. 7 (1967): 1193–1200; Martin Deutsch and the IDS Staff, *The Deutsch Model: Institute for Developmental Studies* (New York: New York University Institute for Developmental Studies, 1968), 11.

6. David Labaree, "The Winning Ways of a Losing Strategy: Educationalizing Social Problems in the U.S.," *Educational Theory* 58, no. 4 (2008): 447–60; David Labaree, *Someone Has to Fail: The Zero-Sum Game of Public Schooling* (Cambridge: Harvard University Press, 2010), 163–221.

7. Sol Cohen, "The Mental Hygiene Movement, the Development of Personality, and the School: The Medicalization of American Education," *History of Education*

Quarterly 23, no. 2 (1983): 123–49; Stephen Petrina, "The Medicalization of Education: A Historiographic Synthesis," *History of Education Quarterly* 46, no. 4 (2006): 503–31.

8. Alice O'Connor, *Poverty Knowledge: Social Science, Social Policy, and the Poor in Twentieth-Century U.S. History* (Princeton: Princeton University Press, 2001), 3–23.

9. Sanford Schram, "In the Clinic: The Medicalization of Welfare," *Social Text* 62, no. 18.1 (2000): 81–107; Joe Soss, Richard C. Fording, and Sanford F. Schram, *Disciplining the Poor: Neoliberal Paternalism and the Persistent Power of Race* (Chicago: University of Chicago Press, 2011), 262–92.

10. See, for example, Kandauda A. S. Wickrama, Rand D. Conger, Frederick O. Lorenz, and Tony Jung, "Family Antecedents and Consequences of Trajectories of Depressive Symptoms from Adolescence to Young Adulthood: A Life Course Investigation," *Journal of Health and Social Behavior* 49, no. 4 (2008): 468–83; Phillip L. Hammack, W. LaVome Robinson, Isiaah Crawford, and Susan T. Li, "Poverty and Depressed Mood among Urban African-American Adolescents: A Family Stress Perspective," *Journal of Child and Family Studies* 13, no. 3 (2004): 309–23; R. N. Bluthenthal, L. Jones, N. Fackler-Lowrie, M. Ellison, T. Booker, F. Jones, S. McDaniel, M. Moini, K. R. Williams, R. Klap, P. Koegel, and K. B. Wells, "Witness for Wellness: Preliminary Findings from a Community-Academic Participatory Research Mental Health Initiative," *Ethnicity and Disease* 16, no. 1, suppl. 1 (2006): 18–34; Tracy Vericker, Jennifer Ehrle Macomber, and Olivia Golden, "Infants of Depressed Mothers Living in Poverty: Opportunities to Identify and Serve," August 2010, http://www.urban.org/uploadedpdf/412199-infants-of-depressed.pdf; Brandon Vick, Kristine Jones, and Sophie Mitra, "Poverty and Severe Psychiatric Disorder in the U.S.: Evidence from the Medical Expenditure Panel Survey," *Journal of Mental Health Policy and Economics* 15, no. 2 (2012): 83–96.

For a sample of media items, see Andrew Solomon, "A Cure for Poverty," *New York Times*, May 6, 2001; "Depression May Underlie 'Transmission' of Poverty," Reuters, January 7, 2009; Donna St. George, "Study Links Poverty to Depression among Mothers," *Washington Post*, August 26, 2010.

Index

Absent fathers, 40, 42, 48, 125, 160, 161, 166

Absurd Healer, The (Dumont), 162–63

Adaptive behavior, 114

Adoption, 13, 65, 124

Aerospace Medical Laboratory, 4

African Americans: antipoverty measures and, 30, 39, 174; childhood nutritional deficiencies and, 48–49; children's speech and, 38, 54–55, 72; compensation proposal for, 158, 159, 165–66, 168; compensatory education and, 110–11, 162, 165, 166; cultural deprivation theory and, 8, 16, 38–44, 50, 54–55, 58–59, 65, 74, 75, 81, 98, 110, 160, 173; cultural heritage of, 39, 58–59, 173; culture of poverty and, 37–38; de facto segregation and, 105, 113, 134–35, 141; deprivation theory applied to, 5, 6, 8, 12, 32, 66, 74, 86, 109–11, 123–24, 157–60, 172–73; differences argument and, 62–73; early childhood educational programs for, 1, 22, 76, 77–86, 132–33; educational inequality and, 62–63, 98, 133–39; empowerment program for, 96–98, 110; Head Start participation and, 109–10; infant intellectual disability prevention programs and, 130, 132; influx into cities of (*see* Inner cities); intelligence theories about, 62–73; juvenile delinquency and, 86–87; Kerner Commission recommenda-tions for, 165–67; language use and, 38, 50, 53, 54–55, 58, 59, 60, 72, 166, 170, 173; limited expectations for, 62; male unemployment and, 161, 164, 166; matriarchy and (*see* Matrifocal family structure); "mild mental retardation" disproportionate diagnosis and, 9, 112, 113, 121, 123–24, 133, 139, 140–41, 173; motherhood images and, 42; Moyni-han Report on, 8, 41–42, 43, 162, 166; racial isolation theory and, 105–6; reading materials for, 81–82; relative deprivation and, 157–58, 165; school desegregation educational benefits for, 105; segregation's effects on, 69, 160, 165, 166–67; sensory deprivation and, 8, 79, 85–86; separation from mother and, 22–23; special education placements of, 13, 135, 138, 139, 140–41, 174; structural deprivation and, 158; test score gap and, 38, 62–65, 69–73, 104, 105–6, 136, 170; urban riots and (*see* Race riots); verbal test scores of, 72; well-meaning liberal stereo-types of, 170; white backlash and, 67; youth groups and, 163–64. *See also* Civil rights movement; Low-income homes; Racism

African American Vernacular English (AAVE), 58–59

Aid to Families with Dependent Children Act, 30

Ainsworth, Leonard, 12

148, 162, 170; infant relationship with, 12–13, 16, 18, 24, 27, 43–45, 65, 66, 70; intellectual development role of, 70; low-income nutritional misinformation and, 48–49; matrifocal family structure and, 8, 40–44, 48, 160, 161, 166, 173; as mediators of all forms of deprivation, 26–28; mentally retarded, 130, 131; middle-class norms and, 7–8, 28, 36, 40, 42, 44–45, 120, 124, 129, 169; racialized images of, 42; stereotypes of middle- and lower-class, 36, 50, 53; three-stage preschool program for, 95. *See also* Working mothers
Mother-substitutes, 10, 124; "professionalization" of, 24. *See also* Day care
Motor deprivation, 18
Moynihan, Daniel Patrick: Head Start evaluation report and, 107–8; *On Understanding Poverty* (ed.), 47; *The Negro Family* (Moynihan Report, 1965), 8, 41–42, 43, 162, 166
Murfreesboro (Tenn.), 77–80
Murphy, Lois, 26, 27, 28, 49, 51, 124, 132

Naked City, The (film), 143
Names: teaching of, 84, 85, 101
National Advisory Commission on Civil Disorders (Kerner Commission), 9, 142, 152–68, 170; final report/recommendations of, 165–67; members of, 152–53
National Association for the Advancement of Colored People (NAACP), 138, 139, 152
National Association of Retarded Children, 116
National Institute of Mental Health (NIMH), 3, 80, 87, 89, 104, 153; intellectual disability intervention programs, 128, 132; Kerner Commission investigation and, 157–58, 161, 164; mass violence research funding by, 157–58; physical environment/

mental health relationship research and, 144–45; "Social-Cultural Aspects of Mental Retardation" (1968 conference), 125–26
National Institutes of Health, 3
National Laboratory on Early Childhood Education, 136
National Organization of Women, 33
National Student Association, 95
National Vitamin Foundation, 100
Native Americans, 66–67
Natural environment, 143, 145
Nature vs. nurture debate, 8, 38, 62–73, 93, 140. *See also* Environmental deprivation; Heredity
"Negro American Intelligence" (Pettigrew), 64
Negro Family, The (Moynihan Report), 8, 41–42, 43, 162, 166
Neurological development. *See* Brain
New Nursery School (Colorado), 103
Newsweek (magazine), 86–87
New York City: early childhood cultural enrichment programs, 76–80; Genovese murder, 142; Lower East Side community action program, 8, 77, 80–93; race riot, 152; strained African American–Jewish relations, 97. *See also* Harlem
New York Daily News, 96
New York Times, 78, 118
New York University School of Education, 81
Niemeyer, John, 95
Nimnicht, Glendon, 104
Nixon, Richard M., 8, 12, 47; day care and, 30–31, 32, 33–35; Head Start and, 34, 35, 107–8; white backlash and, 67
Nobel Peace Prize, 158, 159
"Non-Culture of Poverty, The" (Schorr), 46
Nonhuman Environment in Normal Development and in Schizophrenia, The (Searles), 150
Nonstandard English, 55, 58–60

STUDIES IN SOCIAL MEDICINE

Nancy M. P. King, Gail E. Henderson, and Jane Stein, eds., *Beyond Regulations: Ethics in Human Subjects Research* (1999).

Laurie Zoloth, *Health Care and the Ethics of Encounter: A Jewish Discussion of Social Justice* (1999).

Susan M. Reverby, ed., *Tuskegee's Truths: Rethinking the Tuskegee Syphilis Study* (2000).

Beatrix Hoffman, *The Wages of Sickness: The Politics of Health Insurance in Progressive America* (2000).

Margarete Sandelowski, *Devices and Desires: Gender, Technology, and American Nursing* (2000).

Keith Wailoo, *Dying in the City of the Blues: Sickle Cell Anemia and the Politics of Race and Health* (2001).

Judith Andre, *Bioethics as Practice* (2002).

Chris Feudtner, *Bittersweet: Diabetes, Insulin, and the Transformation of Illness* (2003).

Ann Folwell Stanford, *Bodies in a Broken World: Women Novelists of Color and the Politics of Medicine* (2003).

Lawrence O. Gostin, *The AIDS Pandemic: Complacency, Injustice, and Unfulfilled Expectations* (2004).

Arthur A. Daemmrich, *Pharmacopolitics: Drug Regulation in the United States and Germany* (2004).

Carl Elliott and Tod Chambers, eds., *Prozac as a Way of Life* (2004).

Steven M. Stowe, *Doctoring the South: Southern Physicians and Everyday Medicine in the Mid-Nineteenth Century* (2004).

Arleen Marcia Tuchman, *Science Has No Sex: The Life of Marie Zakrzewska, M.D.* (2006).

Michael H. Cohen, *Healing at the Borderland of Medicine and Religion* (2006).

Keith Wailoo, Julie Livingston, and Peter Guarnaccia, eds., *A Death Retold: Jesica Santillan, the Bungled Transplant, and Paradoxes of Medical Citizenship* (2006).

Michelle T. Moran, *Colonizing Leprosy: Imperialism and the Politics of Public Health in the United States* (2007).

Karey Harwood, *The Infertility Treadmill: Feminist Ethics, Personal Choice, and the Use of Reproductive Technologies* (2007).

Carla Bittel, *Mary Putnam Jacobi and the Politics of Medicine in Nineteenth-Century America* (2009).

Samuel Kelton Roberts Jr., *Infectious Fear: Politics, Disease, and the Health Effects of Segregation* (2009).

Lois Shepherd, *If That Ever Happens to Me: Making Life and Death Decisions after Terri Schiavo* (2009).

Mical Raz, *What's Wrong with the Poor?: Psychiatry, Race, and the War on Poverty* (2013).

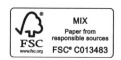